❧ YIN ❧

yoga

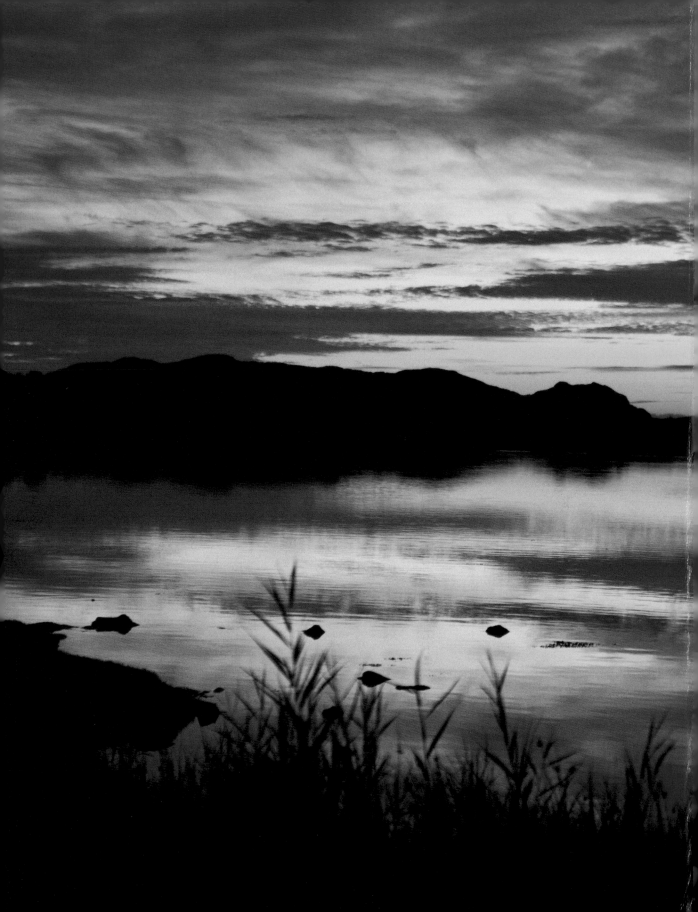

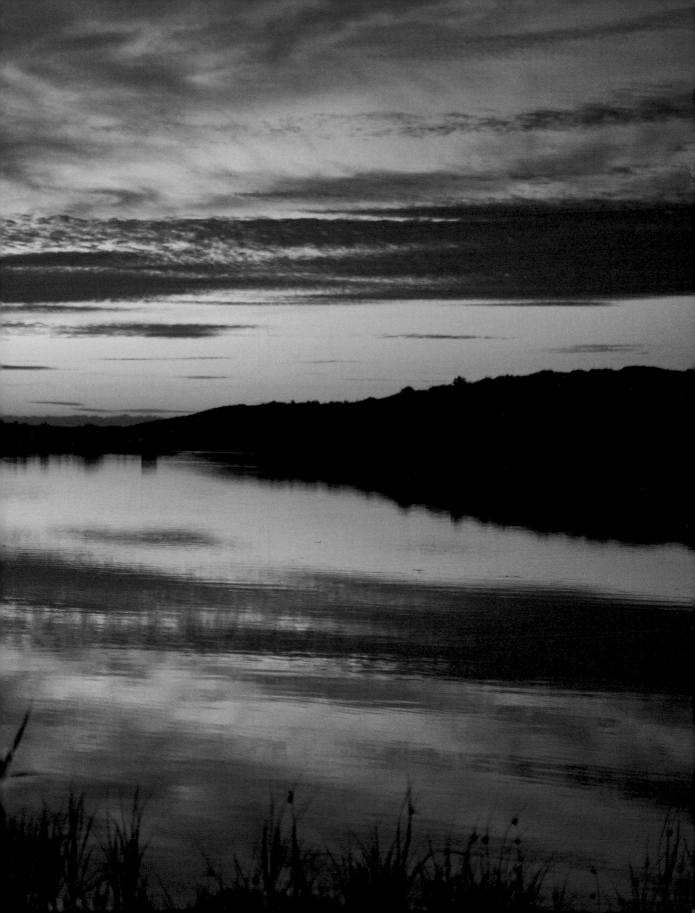

☙ YIN ❧

yoga

AN INDIVIDUALIZED APPROACH TO BALANCE, HEALTH, AND WHOLE SELF WELL-BEING

ULRICA NORBERG

Foreword by Yogiraj Alan Finger
Photographs by Sebastian Forsman

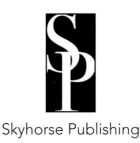

Skyhorse Publishing

Library of Congress Cataloging-in-Publication Data

Norberg, Ulrica.
 Yin Yoga : an individualized approach to balance, health, and whole self well-being / Ulrica Norberg ; photography by Sebastian Forsman.
    pages cm
 ISBN 978-1-62636-395-3 (hardcover : alk. paper)
 1. Yin Yoga. 2. Well-being. I. Title. II. Title: Yin Yoga.
 RA781.73.N67 2014
 613.7'046--dc23
                            2013047289
Printed in China

Important Note:
If you are unsure regarding your health status or if you have any imbalances you might think are affected through yoga practice, please seek advice from a doctor or professional physical therapist before embarking on this practice. This book is by no means a substitute to an experienced yoga teacher who can see your needs and can support you in your practice.

TABLE OF CONTENTS

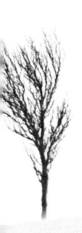

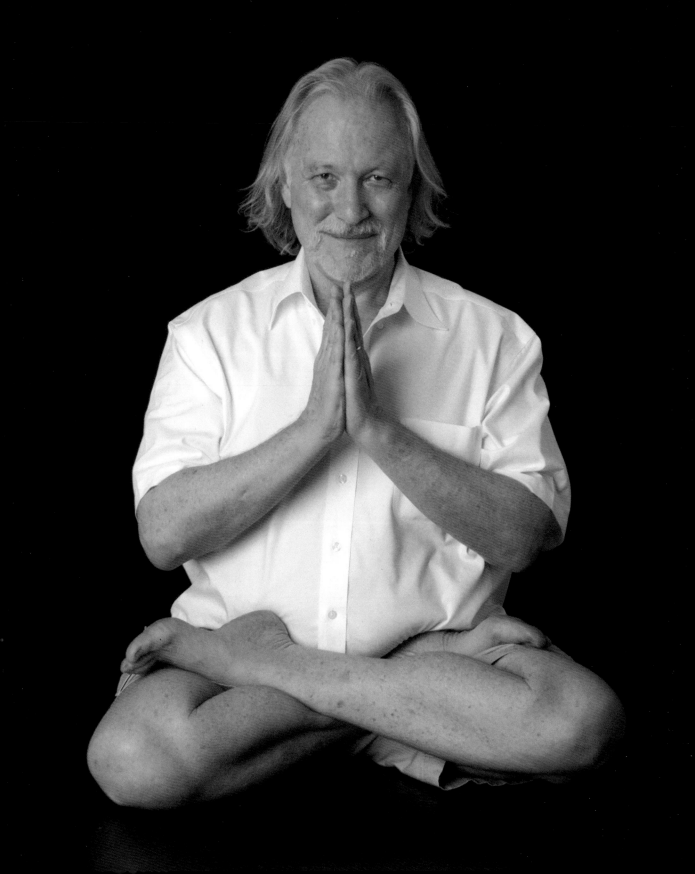

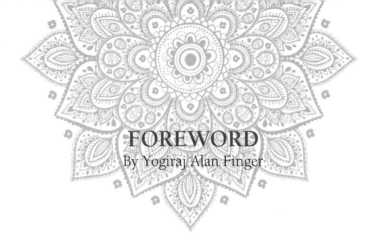

FOREWORD
By Yogiraj Alan Finger

Through her experiences of life in many ways and long-term studies of Yin Yoga, Ulrica has come across a brand new concept of Yin Yoga that I am very pleased to have had a part in by encouraging her and developing this concept with her. I have contributed with my guidance, experience, and expertise, and I fully support this amazing growth.

In our many talks and conversations, Ulrica started to tell me about the art and practice of Yin Yoga and her own experience around adding in ISHTA kriyas into her practice. I inquired more, as I had little reference to this approach to yoga. The more she showed and shared with me about Yin Yoga, the more I felt in my own body that this is a phenomenal way of bringing you to yoga's utter goal: meditation. Since you are holding the poses for several minutes, focusing on your breath, it targets the fascia and calms the nervous system. Kriya is the yoga of the subtle body and its integration is what makes Ulrica's practice of yin so unique. It is a perfect vehicle for one to use to attain better health, a richer life, and more overall well-being. It brings us out from a world where we are controlled by the mind and senses and back to our essence. When we experience *yoga*, we are more in tune with what we need to live a life more in balance with the true self and in alignment with the environment around us.

Through the addition of an ISHTA perspective and especially the kriya techniques, I personally believe Yin Yoga will evolve to an entirely new level, as they are the vehicles through which we can connect back to spirit. Kriyas also inherently align the physical and the subtle body so it is the safest way to practice yin. In her practice as well as in this book, Ulrica does it in such a graceful and delicate way.

In the fast, modern times of today, it is so easy to lose track of one's direction, needs, and self-worth, which often translates to a more extroverted (rajasic) life, usually followed by poor health and unhappiness. As yogis, this tendency also afflicts our practice when it becomes a quest for perfection, wants, and urges. The yoga run by the fluctuations of the mind, rather than a yoga practice that focuses on quieting the mind, is feeding our imbalanced patterns rather than coming back to spirit, where one's true health lies.

That is why Hatha yoga is such a powerful tool. But we need both aspects of Hatha; HA (solar) *and* THA (lunar) and, therefore, Yin Yoga is a fantastic tool in integrating the *tha* aspects of our practice so we can build a more balanced practice.

Ulrica shares her background in an open and transparent way, which is refreshing in a yoga book. I believe this book to be a wonderful inspiration and an additional tool for any yogi on the path to a more individually adapted yoga practice.

Hari Om Tat Sat,

Namaste,

Alan Finger

November 2013
New York, New York

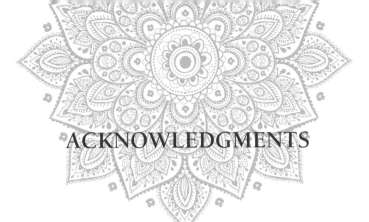

ACKNOWLEDGMENTS

I would like to take the opportunity to express my utmost gratitude to all of you who have supported me throughout this process and to those who have inspired me to keep deepening my understanding of life, the human psyche, yoga, meditation, spirituality, anatomy/physiology/biomechanics, psychology, personal growth, art, and health. I also bow to the art of yoga for showing me the tools to connect to myself to figure out who I am and what works and does not work for me.

To me, life is an exciting avenue to walk on. I see life as a journey on which I get to experience energy in many ways. So thank you to all my ancestors, and to my mom and my dad for granting me life. Also a deep thank-you to my grandmothers, Inga and Lisa; two of the strongest, most inspiring women I have ever met. You have given me so much courage and shown me how to love even when life is challenging.

I would never have been bold enough to write this book if it hadn't been for all the years of practicing yoga and meditation. I bow to my practice since it mirrors so much in myself, showing me where I am in the moment, where I am heading, and what I possess inside. The practice of yoga and meditation holds everything together and awakens me to a fuller existence.

For me, my home and my family are my anchors in life. My biggest supporters are my children, Olivia and Edgar, and my life companion, Magnus. I can never thank you enough for being there with me, every step of the way, supporting me and loving me for me. I love you so much.

I wish to thank my teachers in many areas of study, both academic and non-academic. You all have shown such dedication, devotion, appreciation, and love, and you have shared your knowledge and experience in a personal way.

Some of you have made a deep imprint on my yoga path: Carole Sage, John Sachs, BKS Iyengar, Shri K. Pattabhi Jois, TKV Desikachar, Bryan Kest, Ana Forrest, Chuck Miller, David Swenson, Patricia Walden, Erich Schiffman, Seane Corn, John Friend, Anodea

Judith, David Frawley, Donna Fahri, Shri O P Tiwarij, Dr. Vasant Lad, Gary Kraftsow—to name some of you beautiful masters of yoga.

A special thank you to Paul and Suzie Grilley for teaching me Yin and for bringing Yin Yoga into the public eye and for sharing your knowledge, dedication, experience, and beautiful hearts. And to Sarah and Ty Powers—I carry much love for you and I have the utmost appreciation and admiration for your mastery in the yogic arts. Thank you for all that I have learned and keep learning from you all. You inspire me to keep honoring my inner stillness.

Alan Finger—you are one of the most amazing yoga and meditation masters I have met. I bow to your experience, generosity, and serenity, and I appreciate the cowboy in you. Without that courage, none of us students would have the yoga home in the ISHTA yoga tradition the way we have.

And of course I wish to honor all my colleagues and friends in the ISHTA yoga community and the Sadhaka group, and especially Sarah Platt-Finger and Katrina Repka. You girls rock. I love you.

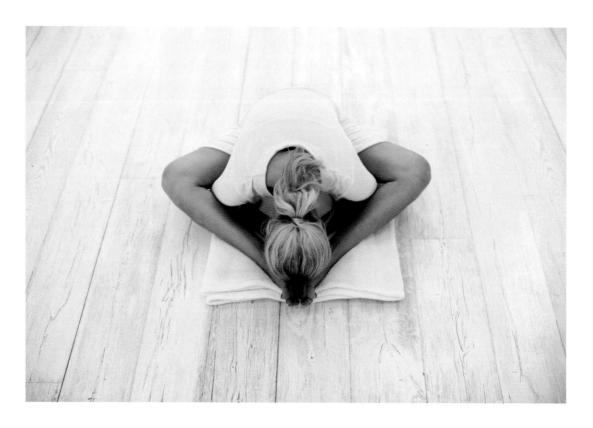

I wish to thank Alan Finger and ISHTA Yoga LLC for granting me the use of ISHTA yoga facts from the Training manuals.

Thank you to Anna Nilsson and the management and staff at the beautiful Asia Spa in Varberg, Sweden, where some of the pictures in the book were taken. You always take such great care of me and show me great support.

Susanne Johansson/Spirit of Maya—you are such a talented woman and I love your fabrics on my body. Thank you for fighting the fight for organic clothing. You bring so much light to us all.

Madeleine and Anders at It's Yoga Studio in Stockholm—you are such amazing human beings. Thank you for being hosts for the ISHTA practice and for taking ISHTA in as a part of the yoga panoply at your studio.

Thank you Sebastian Forsman for doing a fantastic job with the photographs. I salute you and I appreciate our friendship a lot.

My gratitude to Bernie Clark, who has written such great books on the topic of Yin Yoga. Your work is much appreciated by us all.

And thank you to Skyhorse Publishing for giving my story a voice and print and for believing in this book. Abigail and Tony—I bow to you!

Last but not least, to my students. You are the reason I continue to teach and delve deeper into yoga. Thank you so much for your support, dedication, questions, and love. You make me grow as a yogini and teacher.

Hari om tat sat,

Ulrica

September 5, 2013
Stockholm, Sweden

AN INTRODUCTION

"In yoga, if tapas ('heat, or effort') has to do with discipline, commitment, intention to break patterns and purification, Svadhyaya ('self-study') has to do with self-reflection and the journey into who we truly are. Ishvara Pranidhanem ('surrender of results,' or 'relationship with the divine') talks about attitudes and it manifests in the way we handle situations."

—Gary Kraftsow,
Yoga for Self-Transformation

During the last century, we have undergone massive changes in the way we lead our lives. Especially in the Western world, individuals are experiencing higher levels of stress and less physical movement. This is true in both small towns and large cities and for young and old alike. Many European governments have implemented investigations and commissions to study the phenomenon of stress. Some countries have noticed a great increase in people on sick leave due to stress. They have also found that many new illnesses are appearing, all related to psychosocial problems. And every day we hear people talk about depression, exhaustion, and burnout.

Life in the Modern World

Despite advances in medicine, government, and social structure, individuals are experiencing more stress, demands, pressure, and insecurity than ever. Many of us are so absorbed in our highly competitive and fast-paced lives that we are missing out on really living and rarely pay attention to what is happening to us. When we can't keep up any more, we fall. Fall out of health, into despair, and out of our social support systems. We give up, and our bodily systems fail since they are not programmed to keep going twenty-four hours a day. Our systems need to pause and reboot.

If we were to travel back in time to the beginning of the twentieth century and read newspaper clippings and reports from medical doctors and psychiatrists, we'd see a similar phenomenon that these experts called *neurasteny*—nerve weakness due to an undermined and compromised lifestyle. The weakness comes from living your life in a very stressful way, straining the nervous system due to too much physical or mental work, or burdening it with little or no rest. This leads to a lack of energy and motivation. They described it as the "Turn of the Century disease" and claimed it was caused by industrialization. More than a century has passed and we are still suffering from the same symptoms.

The underlying reason for the increase in illnesses like diabetes, migraines, ulcers, skin diseases, hypertension, and digestive imbalances has a lot to do with too much tension in body and mind. Modern medical science is desperately trying to tackle this in many ways, but it can't seem to catch up. This is because the real problem does not lie in the body alone; it has its origins in humanity's changing ideals, in our ways of thinking and feeling. If there is a diffusion of ideals and energy, how can we expect to be in harmony in our bodies and minds?

Our world's biggest problem is not poverty, drugs, fear of war, or hunger. It is tension. All kinds of tension lead to all kinds of imbalances and insecurities. If one knows how to free oneself from tension, one has the solution to one's problems in life. If you are able to balance your tensions, you then automatically learn how to balance your emotions, anger, and passions.

Yogic philosophy as well as modern psychology sum up three basic types of tension that are responsible for all the agonies in modern life. These are *Muscular tension, Emotional tension,* and *Mental tension* (I will cover these in more depth in chapter 2). Through the art and practice of Yin Yoga, these tensions can be progressively reduced. Yin Yoga focuses on the *fascia,* the type of tissue that holds us together. Fascia is the soft tissue component of the connective tissue that provides support and protection for most structures within the human body, including muscle. Fascia is what gives us our form and what makes it possible for us to work our amazing bodies in the ways we do.

The fascia is interlinked with our nervous system and our brain through what's called *tensegrity,* or "The Architecture of life." Tensegrity indicates that the integrity of a structure—in this case, the human body and mind—derives from how all parts are wired together, not how they are stacked. We have fascia everywhere, and our nervous system is enclosed in fascial membranes and continues as nerve sheaths to every corner of the body. Thus different types of strain or tension affect the structure in different ways. From a yogic perspective, you could say we are wired together by spirit, and if spirit is limited in its expresssion, the prana, or life force, will be disrupted, and there will be less freedom for energy to move. Yogis would say that that interrupted prana flow in the mind or body equals less flow in life. Freer flow of prana equals better flow in life. I will talk further about the fascia and its relation to yoga practice, in particular Yin Yoga, in chapter 2.

Vita Contemplativa

In the Middle Ages, a balanced life was referred to as *la dolce vita*—the sweet life—and it consisted of three aspects. First, you needed to have *vita activa*; an active and social life thriving from work, crafts, or trade. Second, you needed good *sleep*. Third, you needed *vita contemplativa*, a contemplative life. This third, more meditative aspect of life was regarded as very important, and it involved time spent alone and in nature. Thomas Aquinas was an Italian Dominican friar and priest commonly known as a natural theologist. His influence on Western thought is considerable, and much of modern philosophy stems from his ideas. He believed that a life led in contemplation is much more valuable than a life full of activity.

Since the start of civilization, we have emphasized the active life (yang) in some cultures and the contemplative life (yin) in others. Now we have the opportunity to explore both and find the appropriate balance between the two. But how do we find time to figure out what we need when everything around us is spinning so fast? Life today doesn't offer natural breaks. We eat lunch on the go and are constantly online or communicating on phones, laptops, or iPads. We may even try to do yoga *while* doing these other things. But to achieve deep relaxation and mental ease, we need a practice where we can turn our senses inward and quiet down. A more yin-based complementary practice is much needed in the life of the modern human and yogi.

The Swedish mysticist Hjalmar Engström describes three steps to stillness:

> *"The first step is to withdraw from the world outside, from everything external, and come into rest. The second thing is to withdraw from your inner desires, even the desire to be still. The third stage is just to be the stillness, which is like a sabbath. This restful sabbath is the source of all things. And when one becomes befriended with this source, it follows her wherever she goes and she becomes free."*

Life Happens

When I was younger, I worried about who I was, what I wanted to do with my life, and where I wanted to live. I yearned for more space and more freedom. I sometimes felt trapped in my emotions and thoughts and by the normatives in Sweden where I lived. I wanted to go out and explore the world. I did what I knew and mastered well: *doing*. I was always doing *more*, always trying harder and never stopped to honor myself and my achievements. Eventually I felt the need to change my perspective, sensing that whatever it was I was looking for would follow. So I did. I left my native Sweden at the age of seventeen to go to the United States as an exchange student.

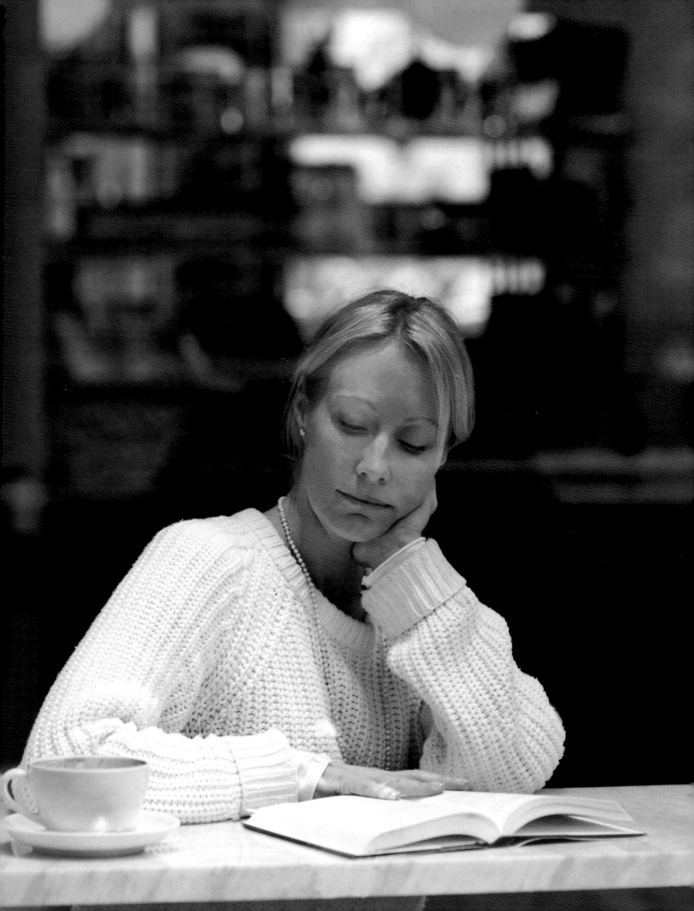

There, I found praise for being me, for what I did and for trying to evolve in more ways than just the academic way. That was very different than what I was used to growing up in Sweden. There, the norm was to be not too much and not too little—just average. At that time in my life, I found that unclear, uninspiring, and not fulfilling. I wanted to explore the edges of existence to know what was out there. Therefore, America was very good for me. I had to work really hard in school, sports, and life, which I loved, and I felt I was recognized for doing so.

I finished high school, went back to Sweden, and got my diploma there as well. In little over a year's time, I was back in the United States again, this time in New York City. I was about to embark on a spiritual journey through the encounter with meditation and yoga and that would change everything. All of a sudden, I found the tool belt I had been looking for to evolve deeper.

Finding a Sanctuary

It was New York and the early 1990s, and I was young and had just gotten out of a relationship that was very destructive. I ran from that man, terrifed, bruised, and battered; he abused me both physically and mentally. I fled as far as I could, to where I could heal and rebuild myself and go on with my life. I wanted to choose *my* life, *my* truth, and *my* path. In the United States I had friends that loved me for me and who inspired me to open my mind, heart, and life to new experiences. And so my spiritual journey began.

My first meditation teacher, a Zen master in the Lower East Village, told me that everyone has a unique potential and capacity. He told me that I should be honored to be me and move through life appreciating what I have rather than chasing after things formed by my imagination and restless mind.

I have always *loved* freedom, searched for it, dreamed of it, and adored it, believing it is a birthright to all humans, so when he said, "Learn how to still the mind and do what you can with what you have and you will be free," it really resonated with me. It still would take me years to develop the confidence and inner security to believe in myself and my capabilities.

The Inquiry Never Stops

I embarked on the path of yoga through studies in Zen Buddhist meditation. Meditation brought me to yoga through Sivananda yoga. Then years followed exploring styles like Jivamuktiyoga, Ashtanga Vinyasa yoga, Poweryoga, Vinyasayoga, Iyengaryoga, and

Anusarayoga. In 2003, I started to study more Viniyoga, yoga therapy, Tantra, and Yin Yoga through many fantastic teachers all around the world.

Many years of studying yoga, meditation, personal growth, being lost, being found, being mindful, being hurtful, doing right, and doing wrong finally got me on the right track. A lot of thanks go to Yin Yoga; a practice that bridges the active with the passive gracefully and was a way for me to start yielding, accepting, and nurturing my spirit. Here I found the piece of the puzzle I was missing; the mind–body connection from a more subtle energy perspective; and a way to move into stillness and heal from tensions of life.

In 2008, I met Yoga Master Alan Finger. After speaking with him for five minutes, I knew he would greatly impact my journey onward. I remember one conversation especially. He said to me, "I see a lot of Shakti[1] in you. Your potential is great but you do not need to do more; rather learn how to integrate what you know with what is you."

Alan is a yoga master from a more traditional background. From a young age he studied yoga, meditation, and Ayurveda with some of the world's most renowed masters from India. Together with his father and teacher, Mani Finger, he put together ISHTA yoga with blessings from their Masters. ISHTA means individualized or "personalized," emphasizing ISHTA's focus on finding the yoga that resonates with the individual's spirit. The second meaning of ISHTA is the acronym Integrated Science of Hatha, Tantra, and Ayurveda. These three principles—*Hatha* (body-mind balance), *Tantra* (energy balance), and *Ayurveda* (Individual balance)—are the three key or "sister" sciences of yoga, and it is through an understanding of applying techniques from these three sciences that the student can blend and find their own practice.

When I first encountered ISHTA yoga, I felt like I was coming home. All my studies and my experiences were honored and deepened and I found a place and space to grow further. In ISHTA yoga, all aspects of yoga is embodied. The yin, yang, and the tao; internal, external, and life. Though ISHTA is my yoga home, I have a lot of admiration and respect for other yoga traditions, since they have all taught me so much.

My take on Yin Yoga in this book is from an individual perspective with a focus from an ISHTA yoga angle.

---

1   Empowerment, feminine creative power

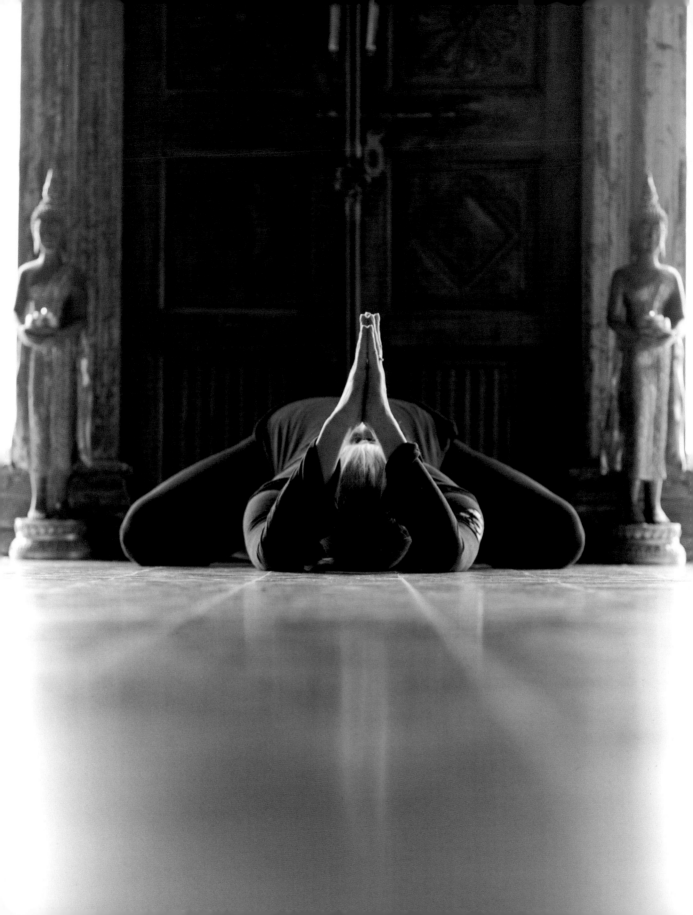

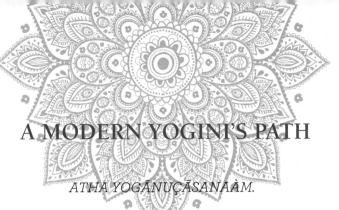

A MODERN YOGINI'S PATH

ATHA YOGĀNUÇĀSANAÀM.

"In the 'now' begins the authentic experience of yoga."

—The Yoga Sutras of Patanjali, Book 1, Sutra 1

We are all battling stress, tension, and mental challenges. I, like most people, have a long list of tasks to accomplish every day and many roles to juggle.

I run my own company; I'm the mother of two small children (with whom spending a lot of time is important to me); I work as a writer, lecturer, coach, and dramatist; I teach yoga and meditation to groups and to individuals; and I conduct trainings and workshops and coordinate various events. But in between, I try just to be still and be *me*. I constantly reflect upon how I can reduce tension and stress in my life. And I have, together with my family, made many conscious decisions to achieve greater space so I can stay attuned to what life has to offer. I want to actually *live* and be a present parent, wife, human being, and yogini and not have my life be solely about tasks and mastering them.

I had IBS for more than twenty years and my husband has ulcerative colitis. Through our experiences living with these imbalances, we realized that these illnesses appeared due to inner tension of different kinds. Living with these issues restricted us so that we could not push as hard as we were used to. Together and separately, we made changes in our lifestyles. Instead of two high achievers with high academic aspirations leading the high life with all that comes with it, we sought a better balance between work, downtime, and family. We lived more moderate lives, with less demanding jobs and fewer possessions. We realized we didn't need to impress anyone—including ourselves—nor try to attain a certain goal in order to be fulfilled in life. We realized we had to make many sacrifices and challenged ourselves in many ways. What strikes me is that when you are trying to break free from the usual way of running a life, and trying to create your own, it costs a lot of energy. And sometimes relationships.

I believe it to be true that one can find one's path and who you really are. But it takes time to find the right tools and learn how to use them. If the tools empower you and give you strength, then you are probably on your way. The thing is, the tools and methods will be slightly different for everyone. It is like the old saying in yoga: "Everyone can do yoga, except the lazy one." To me this means you have to practice, and in your practice you will evolve and understand yourself better.

I have come to the conclusion through my experiences, knowledge, and through the practice of yoga, that all that really matters is health, love, and family. I know it sounds cliché, but I am trying to live this philosophy. My husband and I said to ourselves: "No more talk the talk, now we have to walk the walk. No more ifs, shoulds, and woulds. Lets start living according to all that we have learned."

It is still a process and we do have stress and tension in our lives, but we're well on the way, judging by the fact that we feel better each day. It has been a long and winding road, but the road to spiritual balance is so worth it.

I absolutely love to do nothing, to just be in my Zen, even though I have to fight some mind battles to get there. That is why meditation is so precious to me. When I can really let go and just be in the moment, I become creative, calm, and present. I love to begin my yoga practice calmly and gently, yin-like, then meditate, reground, and then flow into more vigorous, yang-like sequences, before settling again into a softer, yielding mode before *Savasana*. When I honor my practice, the rest of my life becomes a manifestation of that connectiveness and it just runs more smoothly.

Yin Yoga

Yoga means "to yoke" together opposites. That is also what Hatha yoga, the platform for all physical yoga practice indicates—to balance the *ha* (yang) and the *tha* (yin); the solar (doing) with the lunar (being) aspects of the practice. In this sense, our yoga practice should be a blend of yang/out/action/contraction and yin/in/observation/extension to make the whole balanced and to affect our entire health to move towards *homeostasis* (the maintenance of equilibrium). Yangyoga is a more vigorous yoga practice that targets the muscular tissue and through movement creates heat. Examples of yang-based yoga are Ashtanga Vinyasa, Poweryoga, and Anusarayoga.

Through the practice of Yin Yoga, one targets the *fascia*/connective tissue in the body, which makes it a marvellously therapeutic tool for healing bodily, mental, and emotional imbalances. Yin Yoga is most effective when more active forms of yoga or exercise are also practiced regularly.

When you participate in a Yin Yoga class, you will experience mostly seated, supine, or prone poses, and you will stay in the poses, not moving, with your muscles relaxed for long periods of time—up to five minutes, sometimes longer. Staying muscularly passive for long periods of time gently stresses the connective tissue (which gets stiff and immobile with age and through too much or too little use). Yin Yoga poses focus mainly on the lower parts of the body because the abundance of dense connective tissue around the joints in these areas requires extra care and attention.

Yin Yoga is a rapidly growing approach of yoga that has its roots in the United States and was introduced in the late 1980s by martial arts champion and yogi Paulie Zink through his fusion of Taoism and yoga, called Taoyoga. He named familiar poses with different names because they were performed with a totally different objective and effect. Paulie's students approach taoyoga with a new attitude; in order to keep the muscles relaxed with very little resistance over a longer period of time one is able to reach a deeper effect on the connective tissue. This results in greater circulation, less mental strain, and the ability to find relaxation while gently stretching the tissue. The aim is to give the muscle enough time to relax to achieve better elasticity in the connective tissue. We will explore why we would like that to happen and what connective tissue actually is later in the book.

Paul Grilley, Paulie's disciple, evolved Yin Yoga further. Paul's yoga roots stem from Vinyasayoga, Ashtanga Vinyasayoga, and Bikram yoga. He found it difficult to move into meditation after a vigorous flowing yoga practice, which he thought was strange, as he practiced yoga regularly and was very focused. This led him to investigate further. With his training from Paulie Zink and his academic background in anatomy from UCLA under his belt, he continued his studies with Dr. Hiroshi Motoyama, a Japanese scientist whose primary topic is spiritual self and who taught him Chinese medicine, acupuncture, and the energetic system of the chakras.

Years later, Sarah Powers studied with Paul. She was very interested in how the mind and brain work and she brought her master's degree in psychology into her yoga studies, first through styles like Vinyasayoga and Ashtanga yoga. When she met Paul and tried Yin Yoga, she felt like a new world was opening up. Now Sarah fuses Buddhism and mindfulness with Buddhist meditation. Sarah's Yin Yoga style is characterized by mixing Buddhism and Yin Yoga with yangyoga (Vinyasa) sequences.

Finding Yin Yoga

My first encounter with Yin Yoga was in early 2003 when I happened to take a class with Paulie Zink. It was a totally new experience for me. I was asked to explore my limits, both mentally and physically, but not through physical effort or strain. I had to flip the coin and explore the connection between my mind and body from the inside out, not actively, but passively. This was very interesting to me. After class I felt so alive. It was like all my cells were happy, dancing with joy. This made a huge impact on me mentally. I felt much more at ease with myself and others and I recognized the feeling of clarity and alertness that I often had felt after meditation, but this time in all of me, not only mentally. It was like all my cells had been meditating.

I then started to look for Yin Yoga classes but could hardly find any. So I traveled to take classes with teachers who offered Yin Yoga, including Paul Grilley. I felt connected to the way he taught Yin Yoga and his quite scientific and anatomical take on yin and yoga. I bought his book and DVD and continued to practice at home, taking classes when I could. Later I joined his workshops and trainings.

Through him, I discovered Sarah Powers. Her teaching was like sweet music to me; I felt so at home with her teaching style. Since I had been a Zen Buddhist meditator for years, her advocation to bring meditation into the yoga community to a greater extent appealed greatly to me. She is an inspiring woman—so open about herself and who she is is. Her way of incorporating more flowing sequences into Yin Yoga and meditation also resonated with my experiences and studies.

Years of vigorous yoga practice—standing on my head, hands, underarms, in deep backbends, rotations, and forward bends—made me stronger and more alive, but I still did not have a real sense of calm and serenity. I did almost always feel great immediately after Savasana, but often I'd feel restless and anxious a couple of hours later.

Through incorporating a regular Yin Yoga practice, there it was—the connection between the mind being at ease and the body feeling alive and strong. I was amazed that the benefits of my yoga practice lingered much longer. It was as if my body and mind became best friends, allowing the third wingman, spirit, to reveal itself.

Yin Yoga is, to me, a wonderful tool for quieting the riffles of the mind, called *Vrittis*, in order to prepare for meditation. It is also a perfect bridge between meditation and more vigorous yoga practice.

Over the years I have taught Yin Yoga to my students, I've witnessed many different reactions. Restlessness, frustration, irritation as well as emotional releases and bliss—the reaction palate is as wide as life itself. If one moves too strong into the poses, the reactions become wilder. Therefore, a gentler and more yielding inquiry is promoted in this kind of practice and makes you, as a practitioner, gradually release tension and mental restrictions.

I am quite conservative when I teach Yin Yoga, in the way that I pay considerable attention to the anatomy in the beginning of the poses, giving notes on the purpose of the pose and the targeted area. Then I offer variations to find a subtle connection to that area. My experience tells me it is vital to avoid accute pain when one moves into the pose. There is an idea of alignment in Yin Yoga, although from a more subtle body perspective, which I will convey more later throughout the chapters.

My Take on Yin Yoga

One day as I was doing a Yin Yoga practice at home, I automatically felt it was just right to integrate a kriya I had learned from Alan called *Arohan/Awarohan* (explained and demonstrated later in the book) and all of a sudden I was inside my body, in my spirit, with no thoughts hindering me to just be. Also, I was able to keep still longer without effort and I felt that I didn't fall too deep into the poses, which I sometimes do. I am quite flexible and when I suffer from mental tension, then I sometimes go too far in the poses. But not now. So I started to integrate Arohan/Awarohan kriya every time I did yin. After a year of exploring with ISHTA principles in yin, I told Alan and he became interested. Then there was this book to write on the topic on yin. Initially I had a different take on the book, but through this progress in my own practice, and also through sharing it with some close Yin Yoga teacher friends, we noticed the great connection between ISHTA yoga and Yin Yoga principles.

This kriya (vizualisation) technique, also called "the figure eight kriya," revealed in this book, a common technique in the ISHTA yoga system, has never been written down and published in a book. The Tantric kriya techniques are often called "whispering techniques," since they only are conveyed from teacher to student. Traditionally the master gives the disciple the appropriate kriya needed to enhance that student's personal growth and path.

Arohan/Awarohan is a wonderful kriya that helps the practitioner to attain better balance in the practice of Yin Yoga. This, and other techniques, were given to me through my teacher and mentor Yogiraj Alan Finger, masteryogi in the ISHTA yoga lineage, who himself had many kriyas passed on to him by his teachers. When I experimented with it in Yin Yoga, a totally new sensation came about and I noticed how still I became and that my alignment was better.

With this book, I wish to share how I have found better balance in life through the help of these techniques and my thoughts and experiences of Yin Yoga. It is my hope that you will resonate with some of them the way I have.

I have no intention of telling you how to live your life or how to do your yoga. I hope you will find what works for you to heal, feel, and move toward balancing your inside and outside. Take my story and what I share with you in terms of my experience of twenty years of yoga practice and taste it, digest it, and then keep whatever you feel connected to and inspired by.

All I can say is that through practice comes success and progress—not instantly and not in the shapes and forms we expect. Usually happiness reveals itself when we least expect it to and through filters we may not yet be able to grasp with our minds and senses. I am so honored to be able to share some of these techniques with you, and I bow deeply to my teachers Paul Grilley, Sarah Powers, and Alan Finger. You have all contributed so immensly to the yoga community and the world as a whole. Alan has been a wonderful source of information on yoga and fascia, mind, brain, the philosophy, the art of yoga, and what he does best—just being who he is. Through that, he shows how one can be a modern yogi through ancient lineage. Alan encouraged me to write this book and he has been my mentor throughout the process.

It has taken me a little over twenty years of yoga and meditation practice to get me to where I am today. I am finally at a point where I don't want to change in order to "fit in." I fit me and that is enough.

I hope my story will inspire you to weave the yin and tantric aspects of yoga into your life to learn more about yourself and who you are. Yin is a fantastic tool to balance a hectic and demanding life. We need both yin and yang to be whole.

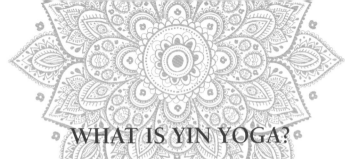

WHAT IS YIN YOGA?

"It's not the size of the dog in the fight, it's the size of the fight in the dog."
—Mark Twain

Yin Yoga introduces us to the natural edges of our beings in a graceful way. If we push our edges or lead a life that is contantly yang, we move into too much yang, burning energy rather than conserving. However, if we draw inward too much or lead too passive of a lifestyle, we start moving away from life and being present, into the past, sliding backward. Too much yin or too much yang creates imbalances. They need to co-exist side by side for us to live our lives in harmony and balance.

Yin Yoga is based on the Taoist concepts of yin and yang, opposing yet complementary forces that can characterize any phenomenon. The earliest reference to yin and yang is in the *I Ching* (Book of Changes) in approximately 700 BC. In this work, all phenomena are said to be reduced to yin-yang.

Yin and yang can be decribed as two variables; they are either on the opposite ends of a cycle, like the seasons of the year, or opposites on a continuum of energy or matter. The opposition is relative and can only be understood through relationships between the two. For example: water is yin relative to steam but yang relative to ice. Nothing is totally yin or yang. Just as a state of total yin is reached, yang starts to grow. This is evident in the Yin Yoga practice, since after you have gotten deep into relaxation and mental stillness in a Yin Yoga pose, the blood circulation increases and you can start to feel heat inside. They constantly transform into each other, just as there can be no energy without matter and no day without light. The classics state that yin creates yang and yang activates yin. This manifests in yoga practice when your breath brings stillness to the mind and you start to flow through the poses. You experience inner heat rather than extensive sweat (that cools your body). This way the metabolism and circulation increases, and your body is able to burn toxins and impurities better.

Yin can be described as stable, immobile, feminine, passive, cold, and downward moving. Yang is depicted as changing, mobile, masculine, active, hot, and upward moving. In nature, a mountain could be described as yin; the ocean, as yang. Within the body, the relatively stiff connective tissue (tendons, ligaments, fascia) is yin, while the pliant and mobile muscles and blood are yang. Applied to yoga, a passive practice is yin, whereas most of today's Hatha yoga practices are yang; they actively engage the muscles and build heat in the body.

If you are accustomed to sweating your way into cool poses, Yin Yoga may at first glance seem too simple, slow, and boring. But this practice of long, passively held floor poses is deeply nourishing and has myriad benefits for any yoga practitioner. After a while of practicing, Yin Yoga is all but boring and easy. It's the opposite. In Yin Yoga, we often say, "Lets move inside and have a look at the interesting things we will find." In Yin Yoga you move inside with the mentality as the observer, not as the force of action where you want to change and go to the edge.

If one does Yin Yoga and aims to push and move away from discomfort, one experiences no effect rather than more frustration and tension and less circulation. With the attitude of the observer, the opposite happens. So when one practices Yin Yoga, it is valuable to have some techniques like breath and visualization to calm the restless and aggressive mind down.

Yang styles of yoga are dynamic and focus on building heat in the body to stimulate, strengthen, and stretch the muscular tissue, and to understand, change, and improve the habitual patterns in the body. Yin is a quiet, more modest form of practice, where we want the muscles to relax to increase circulation in the connective tissue, joints, and organs and to cultivate the ability to yield and observe and accept what is in the present moment.

The most famous symbol of yin and yang is called *T'ai chi,* which means "the highest origin." Society and change are represented in the symbol of light and dark as encircling each other, forming a circle. Yang, symbolized by the white, is at the top, and yin, symbolized by the dark, is at the bottom, with a seed of dark in the light and vice versa.

The circle surrounding the symbol, which in itself symbolizes unity—without beginning and without end—is Tao.

You could say that yin and yang are principles. Yang, whose Chinese character means "the sunny side of the hill," is the principle of activity, and yin means "the shady side" and represents the principle of reflection. Yin represents that which constricts and moves inward, that which remains still. Yang is all that is creative and generating, evolving and expanding, moving. In the body, yin is represented by fascia, and yang by muscular tissue.

Relative levels of yin and yang are continously changing. Normally this is a harmonious fluctuation, but when yin or yang are out of balance they affect each other, and too much of one can weaken the other.

There are four possible stages of imbalance:
1. Excess of yin
2. Excess of yang
3. Deficiency of yin
4. Deficiency of yang

This means that a person can be out of balance in different ways, and the proper thing to do is to add the opposite gradually and through the art of breathing.

An Ancient Practice
The practice of holding yoga poses for long periods of time has always been a significant part of traditional yoga practice, both in the Hatha yoga tradition of India and in the Taoist yoga tradition of the greater China area. Some regard Yin Yoga to be the oldest form of Hatha yoga, since it is an effective method of physical and energetic conditioning for prolonged meditation, which was the principal concern of ancient yogic practitioners. In classical Hatha yoga, some asana were described as Raj asana—seated and reclined meditative poses held passively for longer periods of time.

Nineteenth-century schools of Hatha yoga also advocated holding some poses for relatively long periods of time. For example, BKS Iyengar recommends holding the Supta Virasana asana for 10–15 minutes. Taoist yoga practices from China also included yin-style poses in the Taoist system of "Internal Alchemy"—practices for the purpose of improving health and longevity.

Techniques for stretching of this type have been practiced for centuries as part of Daoist Yoga, which was sometimes known as Dao Yin. Taoist priests taught this knowledge, along with breathing techniques, to Kung Fu practitioners beginning two thousand years ago to help them fully develop their martial arts skills. The intention was to become more flexible and strong mentally, and the path was to go through the body. In Yin Yoga, one learns to let go and allow the body's natural interaction with gravity to stretch the tissues, rather than consciously manipulating one's alignment to achieve a deep stretch. When poses are held for a longer period of time with no effort given to going deeper, reaching further, or searching for results, we practice awareness, contemplation, and reflection. The attention moves inward and allows us to be aware of the thinking patterns we hold within and how they create different currents in our being.

In Yin Yoga, we focus mainly on the lower parts of the body, especially the groin, legs, hips, pelvis, lower back, and spine. Yin is more the lower body, whereas the upper body is more yang. However, there are poses that also work with areas around the stomach and thoracic.

The Inner Workings of Yoga

Some examples of yin and yang:

YIN	YANG
Cool	Heat
Night	Day
Expanding	Contracting
Subtle	Apparent
Earth	Sky
Autumn	Spring
Dark	Bright
Feminine	Masculine
Low	High

Everything in the manifest world can be described as either yin or yang, depending on its primary function and its relation to something else. When we talk about the body, the organs and the legs are closer to the nucleus and can therefore be considered as more yin, while the muscles and the skin are closer to the surface, making them more yang.

Yin and Yang and the Human Body

The front of the body is softer and more vulnerable (yin). The back contains the spine that holds the ribs, which offer protection. When one crouches, the back recieves the sun (yang) and the front faces the earth (yin), which is in shaded and protected. Most of the yang channels flow on the back of the body and protect the body from pathogenic factors. The yin channels flow along the front of the body. Also, below the waist is closer to earth, and is therefore yin. The upper body and head are closer to heaven, and are therefore yang. Through yoga, we balance the front and back, up and down, and the different sides.

Tantric yogic philosophy distinguishes between *the physical body, the subtle body,* and *the causal body.* The subtle body corresponds to what we would call the pysche or mind. It is attached to an individual throughout his or her embodiments in life. The causal body contains karma through which we experience the world and how the world keeps working in cycles. At the material level, we experience the body as separate from its environment. In the higher levels of existence, the boundaries between body and environment become blurred and coexist with the universe. In other words, at the highest level of existence, we literally *are* the world. Tantric philosophy teaches us that if we change our own karma or consciousness, we affect the universal karma or consciousness. Tantra is committed to the idea that we are all part of a larger whole. Thus, in concert with all other beings, we ourselves are responsible for the world we inhabit. Together we create and maintain it.

Although yoga results in overall balance, we carry our individual patterns into our yoga. So if we wish to heal from the inside out, we need to mind our alignment, the relationships between opposites in the body. Therefore, form and content need to be in balance to increase the overall health of a person. A yogi would call the form *prakriti* (matter or nature) and the content *purusha* (spirit or pure conciousness). If we balance the opposites of yin and yang, we balance praktiti (physical) and purusha (subtle)—the forces that make up our form. When we are in balance, yin and yang are in balance.

The Three Principles of Nature

In yogic philosophy, the principle of balance in our nature, prakriti, is illustrated by three states, or tendencies, of energy—Gunas, known as rajas, tamas, and sattva. Rajas (preservation) is activity, tamas (inertia) is passivity, and sattva (creation) is a balance between the two, often described as light and harmony.

According to the text *Yoga Vasistha,* people who are of a sattvic nature and whose activities are mainly based on sattva will tend to seek answers regarding the origin and truth of material life. With proper support they are likely to reach liberation. Rajas is associated with concepts of energy, activity, ambition, and passion; so depending on how it is used, it can result in an extroverted life. Tamas is commonly associated with inertia, darkness, and insensitivity. Souls who are more tamasic are considered imbued in darkness and lead an introverted life.

These are the three forces that exist in nature to manifest energy, similar to the neutron, proton, and electron of the atom. The gunas are the principal building blocks of nature; they bind the individual self to the body by activating the five elements (earth, water, fire, air, and space) and are brought to life by spirit. So if we learn techniques to come into a sattvic state, yin and yang are properly and automatically balanced.

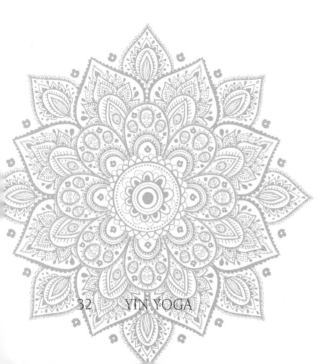

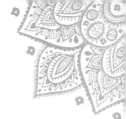

Yin Yoga and the Mind

"Don't lose the mind; use the mind."
—Alan Finger

Before I started doing meditation and yoga, I identified closely with my thoughts and feelings. Today, I have learned to view them more as patterns and reactions coming from my mind and soul. In looking closely at them in meditation, I learn a lot about myself in the now and how I function; and I begin to see what takes me out of balance and out of reach of myself.

Most people get stuck in habitual thought patterns, ways of responding to and acting on events around them, and identification with mental and emotional content. Yin Yoga is a more mindful practice where one can look at and relate to reality and understand one's relationship to it. Paying attention to something can be done in several ways.

The practice of Yin Yoga creates understanding, both of our current condition and of the reluctance or avoidance of being in what we perceive as negative or unpleasant experiences.

Being consciously present means paying attention in the present moment, noticing what is happening both inside and outside when it occurs, and noting thoughts, feelings, and physical sensations without judging or evaluating any part of the experience contained in the present. It is to live your life without being controlled by memories of the past or projections of the future. Life is always here and now.

Buddha described eight conventional attitudes that dominate our mind, which act as fuel for our behavior. They are called the eight worldly dharmas and are described in four pairs of opposites. What we unconsciously or consciously do every day is to swing between these two columns, trying to remain in what we want and avoid what we do not want. Similar divisions can also be found in Patanjali's text *Yoga Sutra*.

What we want:	What we do not want:
Pleasant experiences	Painful experiences
Praise	Criticism
Recognition	Disgrace
Gain	Loss

When the relationship between our desires and our aversions is not examined, the feeling of not being satisfied in life is a constant companion. By questioning and examining our relationship with these eight worldly dharmas, we can begin to understand the common denominator: the inescapable truth that everything changes.

Through a more mindful practice like Yin Yoga, we can learn to live with both pleasant and unpleasant experiences, both gain and loss. Without trying to get rid of or deny difficult experiences, we learn to be open to vulnerabilities without averting the direct experience of them. Through conscious attention, we investigate for ourselves the liberating opportunity to stop struggling with pain, criticism, shame, and loss. We attain curiosity and acceptance and learn to relate to all of life's experiences, without categorizing them as good or bad. They are simply experiences that come and go.

The first step to attaining a more relaxed and neutral (sattvic) mindset is to learn how to quiet the *vrittis*—the restlessness of the mind (the amplitude of the brainwaves)—through the practice of yoga in relation to meditation.[2]

> *"To perceive meditation we need to understand the relationship between Mind and Spirit. Spirit is experienced when our consciousness is not fragmented by mind."*
> —Alan Finger

The vrittis can be understood as waves on a lake or an ocean. The waves come from the wind blowing (the underlying turbulence behind our thoughts; the unconscious). If we can stop the wind from blowing (calm the unconscious) then the lake becomes calm and reflects the sky and stars (spirit). If the lake is wild, you cannot see anything. This is why a daily practice is so utterly important. The daily yoga and meditation *Sadhana* (the practice) trains the brain and nervous system to stay present without reacting to

---

2   ISHTA Yoga Teachers' Training Manuals.

everything around you. You train the brain like you train a muscle. The more you practice, the more skilled you will become. From a yogic point of view, it is very necessary for a yogi to connect to spirit (all that is you) every day. Then if there is a storm, you will still remember how it was before the storm and what's behind the clouds, and you won't fall over from your reactions, which will make you crazy.

These thought patterns (vrittis) are mastered (nirodhah: regulated, coordinated, controlled, stilled, quieted) through practice (abhyasa) and non-attachment (vairagya) to the results (bhyam tan nirodhah).
—Yoga Sutra: 1:12

To be a yogi, you just have to practice yoga regularly. The yoga will do the rest. Becoming a yogi doesn't mean giving up the old you and becoming someone else. However, things that are not serving you well may fall away. As you practice yoga, you move toward the more intuitive, less fragile you. On the other hand, being a yogi doesn't mean you don't have problems; you just have more tools for dealing with them. Yoga provides *kaivalya*, or space around your experience that allows you to have perspective regarding your problems and what to do about them.

The demands of Western culture can easily lead to low self-esteem. While there is usually room for improvement, we are all amazing beings just as we are. In a yoga practice we should just get to the mat, work within our limitations, and feel how we detach from all of what inhibits us, rather than get caught up in competitiveness. Just do the practice without looking for some specific result.

Sah tu dirgha kala nairantaira satkara asevitah dridha bhumih.
When that practice is done for a long time, without a break, and with sincere devotion, then the practice becomes a firmly rooted, stable, and solid foundation.
—Yoga Sutra: 1.14

As a tantric yogi, you rely on yourself and what you observe as an individual rather than on dictates and rituals. You come into contact with your highest self through meditation and act according to your intuition and intelligence through clarity. This makes shoulds and should nots superfluous. You gain the ability to move toward a more predominantly sattvic (harmonious, intelligent) state rather than constantly being at the extremes of rajas (passion, energy) or tamas (inertia, ignorance).

There is a misperception that an "enlightened yogi" is passively accepting of all circumstances and will not care how she is treated or what her circumstances may be. True study and application of your practice will erase many of those misperceptions. For example, there is no sutra stating that the true yogi never says no. Sometimes practicing truthfulness and respect for yourself, others, and a given situation may result in *more* action as you develop clearer boundaries and integrity. This has been my experience. Before yoga and meditation, I had little awareness of my own boundaries and I had never been shown to move inward for answers. I searched on the outside instead and I had such a need for affirmation and acceptance that I never said no. For me, it took many years of practice and life lived to move more into sattva guna—to a more centered positioning in myself where I could speak of my needs. This spiritual maturity gave me the ability to better accept different situations, to focus better on tasks, and to not get as emotionally involved as I used to be. [3]

From a tantric point of view, our conciousness, *citta*, has two functions: the lower mind and the higher mind.

THE LOWER MIND

The lower mind is composed of our five bodily senses, or *Indriyas* (touch, smell, taste, vision, and sound), and our intellect, *Buddhi*. Together they form our reactions. Buddhi, together with memory (*Smrti*), the I-ness or sense of self (*Ahamkara*), and perception (*Manas*), creates the yogi's strength and motivation to move through *Dukha* (pain and unfulfilled desire), *Avidya* (ignorance), *Maya* (illusion), and *Asmita* (ego) to reach the higher mind.

THE HIGHER MIND

The higher mind consists of the *Atman*, the soul derived from spirit. This is the essence of being connected to spirit, and once you reach this state of consciousness you discover insight—the ability to let go and be guided by spirit, your intelligence.

Yin Yoga is a fantastic practice in which to apply ISHTA techniques like *pranayama* (breathing exersices) and *kriyas* (visualization) to connect to the subtle body and the higher mind. Yin Yoga is very much a yoga practice for the nervous system and the brain in that it reduces tension and stress, and balances the mind to reach our higher self.

---

3   ISHTA Yoga Teachers' Training Manuals.

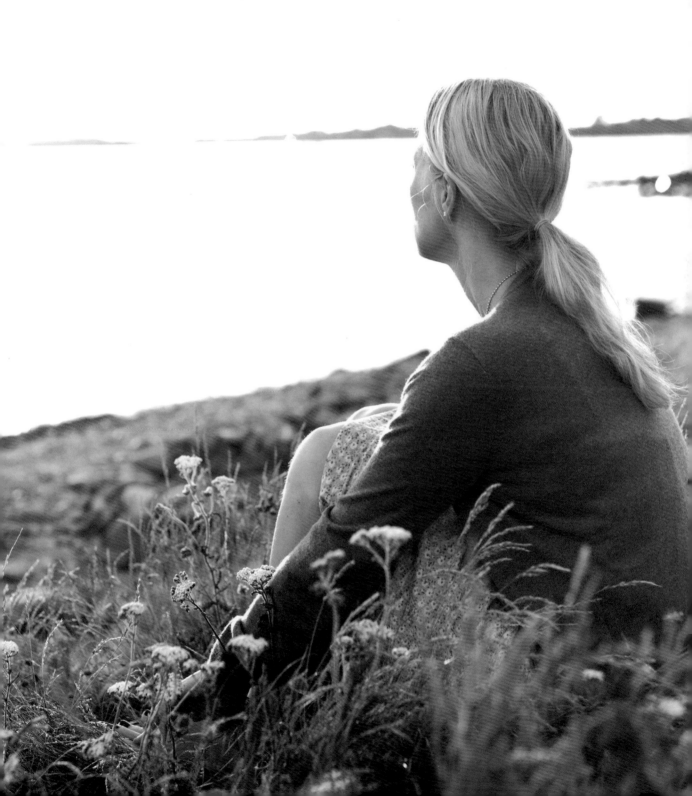

Therefore, Yin Yoga can be a wonderful complementary practice to any yang-oriented practice (flowing yoga, running, or weightlifting to name a few).

The Interaction of the Inner Energy

"If we all worked on the assumption that what is accepted as true is really true, there would be little hope of advance."
—Orville Wright

The main objective of hatha yoga (physical yoga), is to create an absolute harmony of the interacting activities and processes of energy, mind, and physical body. In Hatha yoga, *ha* represents prana, the vital force, and *tha* represents mind, the mental energy. Therefore hatha yoga is about the union of pranic (prana shakti) and mental forces (manas shakti). When this occurs, the awakening of higher conciousness happens in the individual. Every object in the universe, from the atom to the star, is composed of these two energies. When they interact with each other, creation happens, and when they are separated they move back to their source and creation is dissolved. This is described as the total annihilation of matter.

All matter in this creation is alive and conscious. Therefore, everything has potential and everything is alive. In yoga, consciousness and life are known as purusha and prakriti; in tantra, they are named shiva and shakti. In Hatha yoga, they are named pingala and ida; in taoism, as yang and yin; and in physics, as energy and matter. They have differnet names in different times and philosophies.

The dualities of matter and energy can be translated to the human nature. We have a physical body but we also have a subtle counterpart, too. So what happens on the inside when you think? What happens inside you when one thought results in the next? In yoga, one should always keep in mind that the body, mind, and the spirit are not three; they are one. At one level you see the body and at another you see it as the mind. The spirit is never different from the body and vice versa. They are one.

The *prana shakti* and *manas shakti* are usually in an unbalanced and unharmonized form in us. One of them is usually predominant over the other, creating imbalances in mind, body, and spirit. Due to this imbalance, physical disease or mental diseases manifest. The techniques of yoga like asana (body posture), pranayama (the art of breathing properly), and kriyas (to focus the mind) are to bring these into better harmony and learn how to calm the nervous system and cleanse the body from toxins.

The nervous system needs to be trained since it is the carrier of impulses through the sensory and motor channels. For an uninterrupted flow of energy to pass throughout the body, it is vital that you move into *pratyahara*, or sense withdrawal. If you don't, then it is hard to meditate. Pratyahara is the bridge between the physical/mental and the subtle body awareness and of spirit.

The first tool to apply to move into pratyahara is learn how to breathe properly and, through breath, to start to move and direct energy, or *pranayama*.

The subtle body is the energetic mold of the physical body. It is more accessible to the mind and consious control. On a subtle level, change is somewhat fragile and demands powerful intention. Once change on a subtle level has filtered down on a physical level, it tends to be more stable. This means it is difficult to make and maintain change purely on a physical level. For example, a person can exercise and eat properly and still be affected by ill health.

Tantra[4] has evolved its own form of therapy, little known in the West still. It is based on the self-purification not only on a physical and mental level, but also on an energetic level. Physical purification has been greatly elaborated through Tantric yoga. Mental purification consists primarily through meditation and visualization. And energetic purification, which is the forte of Tantra, is carried by means of visualization and breath control (aka *prana* energization and harmonization). Prana is on the subtle level what breath is on a physical level. By aiming to remove energetic blockages ad correct damage on a subtle level, tantric practitioners prevent physical disease and mental imbalance.

"Whatever controls Prana controls the mind and whatever controls the mind controls Prana."
—Hatha yoga Pradipika 4. 21

Breath Carries Everything
Breath is a life force; we begin our life with a breath and we end it with a breath. The breath, body, and mind all work together. If one of these is agitated, the others will follow. If one is calm, the others will follow.

From the breath, we receive oxygen, which nourishes the blood, organs, and cells, and *prana*—life force—travels on oxygen. Through breath, our physical body is linked to the mind, and the mind to the life force, prana. The breath enhances the mind–body connection, so when we start to cultivate the breath, we connect to our higher self.

---

4   ISHTA Yoga Teachers' Training Manuals.

The yogic texts and masters state very clearly that to balance the mind, one needs to control the prana inside. If prana is restless, mind becomes restless and vice versa. The mind is very difficult to control and the more ones struggles, the harder it gets. By practicing pranayama correctly, the mind is automatically stilled. The general idea is that pranayama ought to remove blockages in the autonomic nervous system (ida and pingala nadi) to have the breath run evenly in both nostrils. When the flow is even in both nostrils, your nervous system is in harmony and you move easily into meditation.

The breath is one of only two functions of the body that is both voluntary and involuntary (the other function is blinking). If we can master breath consciously, we can control other functions in the body like heart rate, blood pressure, and breath. Through the breath, we can access the parasympathetic nervous system and activate the relaxation response in the brain, which results in stress reduction for our entire system.

Most people are not breathing to their fullest capacity, which actually means that the nerve cells are not fully activated, which chokes the life force in us. Through conscious breathing, we can mindfully generate more oxygen for the body.

Tightness or stress in the body often creates tightness in the breath. Think of wearing a body suit that is too tight—it is hard to breathe. When your body is tight and tense, you can't breathe fully. You can be tight in your breathing body just like you are tight in your physical body. Some of this is physical strain impinging on the breath volume; some is emotional or mental blockage preventing us from breathing fully.

Our mental condition affects the breath, which in turn affects postural habits. For example, if you are depressed, stressed, or tired, you slouch and cannot breathe fully. This creates tightness in the body. By breathing more fully, one can change one's mental and physical state.

Yoga is a tool to make our unconscious patterns conscious. Through conscious awareness, we are released from our patterns: physical, breathing, mental, physiological. Each one affects the other. Changing the patterns of your breath changes the patterns of your body, your mind, and your life. Breathwork increases freedom in our breathing and freedom in our living. When we liberate ourselves from our patterns, we become more aware of the most subtle aspects of being.

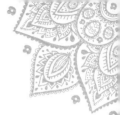

The Full, Complete Breath

One breath consists of four components:

1. *Pooraka*: inhalation
2. *Antar Kumbhaka*: pause/breath retention
3. *Rechaka*: exhalation
4. *Bahir Kumbhaka*: pause/breath retention

As we inhale, the diaphragm lowers for the lungs to expand. The muscles between the ribs, called intercostals, expand and lift the rib cage, and the entire circumference of the abdomen expands. Then on an exhale, the abdomen relaxes, the belly draws in, and the diaphragm releases back up into the chest as a second set of intercostal muscles contracts and returns the rib cage to its starting position.

Observing the interaction of our rib cage and diaphragm, we are reminded of an umbrella. The "umbrella" opens on inhale and closes on exhale. Being conscious of full, complete breathing is our aim while we are practicing yoga.

In the practice of Yin Yoga, it is recommended to use a breathing technique that brings you to pratyahara. You do not want to use a manipulating breathing technique, but a method that brings you to a proper, natural, and deep breath to help settle the mind and calm the nervous system. I recommend the *Full, Complete Breath Exercise*.

FULL, COMPLETE BREATH EXERCISE

To get familiar with this breath, you can do this initial exercise:

Props Needed: One or two towels. If the chin lifts higher than the forehead, place the blanket underneath the head to lengthen the back of the neck. If the lower back is sensitive, place a rolled blanket underneath the knees.

On the inhale:

1. Notice the breath in the chest making the side ribs expand and the top corners of the chest lift up.

2. Feel the floating ribs in the back expand and press down toward the floor, giving you the sense that there is a tiny flotation cushion underneath your middle back.

3. Notice the belly expand slightly.

On the exhale:

  1. Feel the movement begin just below the navel as the belly draws up and inward.

  2. Feel the sides of your rib cage draw inward towards the center of the spine.

  3. Let the shoulder blades softly slide downward on your back.

  4. Allow the rib cage to settle back down to its starting position.

  5. Continue feeling the subtle movements of a full, complete inhale and a full, complete exhale.

It may be difficult to feel all of those subtleties at first. That's fine. The first step toward feeling those dynamics is to *visualize* the movements taking place. Doing that will help draw your senses inward and keep you tuned in to your breathing so you do not drift off in your thoughts. In addition to physiological changes and increases in oxygen, this inward focus is one of the primary benefits of pranayama practice.

The full, complete breath is not an impossibility, no matter how long you have been breathing another way. As babies, we breathed full, complete breaths. We can find our way back there again.[5]

In the Yin Yoga practice, the full complete breath is a marvellous tool that will help you pay attention to what the body is trying to tell you. The breath is also the force that your attention travels on. So when you manage to attain your focus through the breath you then add the kriya, or visualization technique of *Arohan/Awarohan* (soon to be properly introduced and explained), in order to maintain good alignment and also to balance rajas and tamas tendencies in our body and mind. This so your practice can become sattvic and healing/balancing.

Full, Complete Breath and the Body

Full, complete breathing requires balanced posture. Balanced posture begins with the feet if you are standing or, if you are sitting, your sitbones. When standing, place the feet evenly on the ground. When the weight is distributed between the ball and the heel and the

---

5   ISHTA Yoga Teachers' Training Manual.

arches are slightly lifted, then the leg muscles are being engaged correctly to support the weight of the torso. When seated, ground the sitbones down toward Earth and soften the lower back as you slowly lift the sternum up and soften the shoulder blades down. When our torso is freed of trying to hold the body up and when the shoulders are relaxed, then the muscles in the trunk can be free to breathe fully, as they were designed.

When someone walks into a room with correct posture and easy, flowing, complete breaths, that person's poise, self-esteem, and calming presence command your attention. We can learn to find balanced posture and full, complete breathing in a host of different body alignments by practicing the *asanas* taught later in this book.

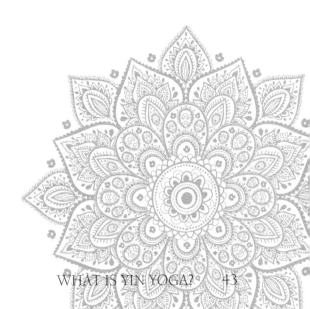

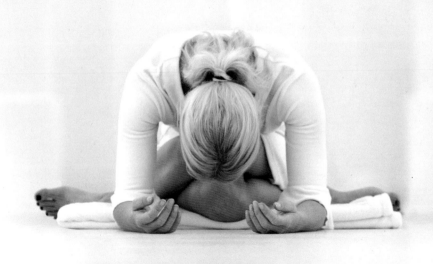

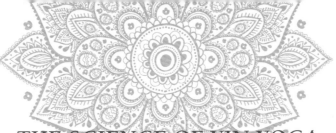

THE SCIENCE OF YIN YOGA

YOGAÇ CITTA VRITTI NIRODHAHA.

"Yoga occurs when the consciousness (citta) is free of modifications (vritti).
Yoga happens in the Now."
—The Yoga Sutras of Patanjali, Book 1, Sutra 2

Yin Yoga's goal, on a physical level, is to target the connective tissue, often also called *fascia.* (Fascia is often defined as a type of connective tissue, existing around and inside everything, giving form.) *Connective tissue* is a generic term for various tissue types in the body. Its functions are to support the body structure, to hold the joints and organs in place, and to transport signals and operating energy. Ligaments, tendons, muscle, cartilage, fascia, and bones are types of connective tissue.

As we age, our connective tissue stiffens, limiting circulation in the body, which then affects the mind and brain. When the brain doesn't get enough circulation and waste products accumulate in the body, the aging process accelerates. Yin Yoga offers us a way to unwind and loosen up, increasing circulation, and detoxifying the body and mind.

Connective Tissue
Connective tissue is different from muscle and needs to be exercised differently. Instead of the rhythmic contraction and release that best stretches muscle, connective tissue responds best to a slow, steady pull. If you gently stretch connective tissue by holding a yin pose for a long time, the body will respond by making the tissue a little longer and stronger—which is exactly what you want.

Although connective tissue is found in every bone, muscle, and organ, it's most concentrated at the joints. In fact, if you don't use your full range of joint flexibility, the connective tissue will slowly shorten to the minimum length needed to accommodate your activities. If you try to flex your knees or arch your back after years of underuse, you'll discover that your joints have been "shrink-wrapped" by shortened connective tissue. In yoga we do three things to the tissues in the body:

1. Compress to move bone to bone. (In backbends, for example, we compress the spine but aim to lengthen the spine first.)
2. Stretch to work with tension. (Forward bends are a good example of this since we stretch the back of the body where we usually store a lot of tension.)
3. Twisting. (All rotation of the spine in poses makes the tissues wrap up against each other which is good for the vitality of the tissues.)

As I mentioned above, connective tissue is often called fascia. It is the more popular word for this amazing tissue in our body, bringing form to all in us. Fascia means ban/bandage in Latin and it needs to be rejuvenated to be strong and healthy. It works like a sponge; when we bring fluids in and massage it, it can release toxins and tension. You can think of a water hose. If you haven't used it for years and flood water into it, its sides might crack and break. Same for fascia. It needs to be used and to have some pressure on it to maintain elasticity.

Connective tissue is one of the four main types of tissue that make up the body: muscle tissue, nerve tissue, epithelial tissue, and connective tissue. These fibrous groups of cells hold together the other types of tissues, including muscles, nerves, and epithelium. (Epithelial tissue is supplied with nerves, but not with blood vessels. Epithelial tissue has many functions, including protection, secretion, selective absorption, excretion, diffusion, and sensation). Connective tissue is made up of a combination of living cells and non-living material known as matrix. It's everywhere in the body, around and between organs and other tissue. It's most concentrated around our joints.

Many people who come into contact with Yin Yoga recoil when you mention that you work with the connective tissue and stretch it. But Yin Yoga is not about stretching the connective tissue; it's about putting gentle stress on it over time to increase elasticity and circulation. For instance, in Yin Yoga we never stretch knees side to side, as the knee is not designed to stretch in that direction. In Yin Yoga we work toward full flexion and extension (bending and stretching), generally working only with the area around the hips, pelvis, and lumbar spine.

Connective tissue is a versatile tissue group. It mainly consists of macromolecules rather than cells. Typically, connective tissue is also an *avascular* tissue; that is, a tissue that lacks blood vessels. The cells of the connective tissue are responsible for defense (white blood cells) and the production of fibers (plasma cells, fat cells, and fibroblasts).
Connective tissue can be divided into groups as follows:

1. *Loose connective tissue/areolar connective tissue.* Loose connective tissue is a mass of widely scattered cells whose matrix is a loose weave of fibers. Many of the fibers are strong protein fibers called collagen and elastin. Loose connective tissue is found beneath the skin and between organs and surrounds muscles, nerves, and blood cells. It is a binding and packing material whose main purpose is to provide support to hold other tissues and organs in place. *Areolar* means that it does not consist of blood. If the skin becomes inflamed, the loose connective tissue is affected.

2. *Adipose connective tissue.* Adipose tissue consists of adipose cells in loose connective tissue. Each adipose cell stores a large droplet of fat that swells when fat is stored and shrinks when fat is used to provide energy. Adipose tissue pads and insulates the animal body. It consists of a significantly higher proportion collagen and therefore has great elastic strength. It is found in the muscles, tendons, and ligaments around the bone joints that should be able to cope with continuous, daily pressures and significant load peaks while weightlifting.

3. *Blood connective tissue.* Blood is a loose connective tissue whose matrix is a liquid called plasma. Blood consists of red blood cells, erythrocytes, white blood cells, leukocytes, and thrombocytes or platelets, which are pieces of bone marrow cell. Plasma also contains water, salts, sugars, lipids, and amino acids. Blood is approximately 55 percent plasma and 45 percent formed elements. Blood transports substances from one part of the body to another and plays an important role in the immune system. This type of connective tissue is available in lymphoid organs such as bone marrow, the spleen, and lymph nodes.

4. *Specialized; collagen connective tissue.* Forms include bone, cartilage, and adipose tissue. As early as the fetal stage, the skeleton forms using compact and tough cartilage. As minerals are stored in the connective tissue, cartilage hardens to bone.

Collagen (from the Greek *colla*, meaning "glue," and *genos*, meaning "descent") is a dense connective tissue, also known as fibrous connective tissue. It has a matrix of densely packed collagen fibers. There are two types of collagen: *regular* and *irregular*. The collagen fibers of regular dense connective tissue are lined up in parallel. Tendons, which bind muscle to bone, and ligaments, which join bones together, are examples of dense regular connective tissue. The strong covering of various organs, such as the kidneys, is dense irregular connective tissue.

Cartilage (from the Latin *cartilago*, meaning "gristle") is a connective tissue with an abundant number of collagen fibers in a rubbery matrix. It is both strong and flexible. Cartilage provides support and cushioning. It is found between the discs of the vertebrae in the spine, surrounding the ends of joints such as knees, and in the nose and ears.

Bone is a rigid connective tissue that has a matrix of collagen fibers embedded in calcium salts. It is the hardest tissue in the body, although it is not brittle. Most of the skeletal system is comprised of bone, which provides support for muscle attachment and protects the internal organs.

The eye wall is also composed of dense, collagen-rich connective tissue that protects the eye's interior and makes sure the eye retains its shape.

Fascination with Fascia

The great Leonardo da Vinci's intricate drawings of human anatomy were ahead of their time, and their detail and accuracy make them a significant contribution to the fields of both the arts and the sciences. Since then, we have seen five hundred years of advances in medicine, so you would think that Western science would have human anatomy pretty well figured out. But it doesn't. Why? *Fascia.*

The medical community regards fascia primarily as a tissue structure that links together all the bones, muscles, nerves, blood vessels, and organs of the body. But the fact is, fascia serves many purposes, such as being involved in movement and the transmission of force. According to new reserach, fascia is regarded as part of the nervous system in that it provides a communication network throughout the entire body.

There are three basic systems associated with fascia: the *articular* (circulation), the *neural* (information process system), and the *myofascial* (anatomy) network. Fascia should also be looked at as a semiconductive communication network in that it is capable of sending nerve signals that communicate with each other throughout its network. This means that the fascia affects the whole body, not just one area or system.

According to the research of the scientists Hiroshi Motoyama and James Oshman, pressure put on the connective tissue during yoga stimulates fibroblasta to produce more hyaluronic acid (HA), which is a primary component of synovial fluids that exist in joints. HA has the property of attracting much water, which is a good electrical conductor. If this theory is accurate, it would explain why Yin Yoga strenghtens the joints and nervous system in the body—it stimulates the production of HA.

The Methodology of Yin Yoga

Since we hold the poses longer in Yin Yoga—breathing and keeping still—blood, nutrients, oxygen, and tissue fluids circulate to dry and compact tissue with poor circulation. At the same time, there is a purging of toxins and increased lymphatic circulation, while fluid accumulation decreases. When there is balance in the circulation of the connective tissue, the body is healthier and the immune system improves.

Yin Yoga techniques increase the blood flow, sending it right out to the very tips of one's limbs, relaxing one's muscles.

Western medical research is now quite clear that connective tissue zones are connected to the autonomous nervous system. If you experience strong mental or physical stress that results in muscles becoming tense, you become dizzy or cold, you experience worse digestion, and so on, Yin Yoga can help you release tension at a rate appropriate to the individual. You could say that Yin Yoga is yoga for our joints and that Yang Yoga is yoga for our muscles. Yin Yoga balances the active and dynamic lifestyle and yoga practice we already have.

With Yin Yoga, one can get more range of motion (ROM) in their joints and open them to a healthy limit. The range of motion in the joints are affected by tension that can come from too much hard exercise, unbalanced breathing and diet, and also from unbalanced compression that usually arrives due to too much sitting, poor posture, and stress.

Yogic philosophy states that prana flows through our joints, so if we want more prana to circulate in our systems, we need to create space in all aspects of our being—in our joints as well as in our spirits. When we can relax and unwind, the circulation increases and our inner and outer balance comes more into place.

There are two principles that differentiate yin practice from more yang approaches to yoga: holding poses for at least several minutes (working toward stillness) and stretching the connective tissue around a joint. To do the latter, the overlying muscles must be relaxed. If the muscles are tense, the connective tissue won't experience the proper stretch.

It is important to aim for varying poses so you move the spine in all its directions to affect the fascia in the legs, pelvis, and spine. The different planes of movement are flexion (forward bends), extention (backbends), lateral flexion (side leaning), and rotation.

Mental Benefits of Yin Yoga

Yin Yoga can be a marvelous tool to learn to be more comfortable in situations we otherwise relate to as difficult or unpleasant. Yin Yoga positions can trigger emotional and psychological challenges. We can learn to relate to these challenges in a new way, and we can see how the once strong reactions may change over time to be not as strong.

Perhaps sensations are as strong, but the way we react to them has changed. You have less resistance to the experience, curiosity and desire emerge, and eventually you can feel and participate in the experience fully as it is. Yin Yoga helps with relieving all kinds of tension and has a positive effect on the nervous system and brain. The brain waves calm down in lower amplitude.

The Relaxation Response

Herbert Benson, professor at Harvard Medical School and founder of the Mind/Body Medical Institute, discovered the so-called relaxation response. His studies have shown that the relaxation response is when metabolism, blood pressure, heart rate, respiration, and muscle tension all decrease, and a slow brain wave—alpha—increase occurs.

Two factors must be present to elicit the relaxation response:
1. The mind is focused on something repetitive (sound, breath, movement)

2. An attempt is made to let go of all other thoughts (this attempt *does not have to be successful*)

This effect can be achieved while practicing yoga, running, prayer, knitting, walking, meditating, pranayama, visualizations, etc.

Upon inducing the relaxation response, the physiology of the body is the opposite of a stress response. This relaxed state has a profound healing effect. You don't have to feel relaxed—in fact, you can feel agitated and restless while trying to let go of all your thoughts and still induce the relaxation response. The calming effects are more dramatic and faster than any other means—even sleep.

After four to five hours of sleep, oxygen consumption levels are at 8 percent less than when in a waking state. The relaxation response lowers oxygen consumption 10 to 17 percent in the first three minutes. The relaxation response nullifies (to a certain extent) the action of noradrenaline (the hormone that increases heart rate and blood pressure) so that the body does not react as radically to mildly stressful events.

The benefits of relaxation are cumulative, protecting you from stress long after practicing these techniques. The clearing of the mind can reprogram the patterns and negativity of the mind. On a psychological level, it is about being—not doing. For many of us, this is the first time we have had the experience of having no goals, no place to move toward, but instead just being and doing nothing. When we taste this state of being, our mind clears, our hearts open, and our sense of self expands.

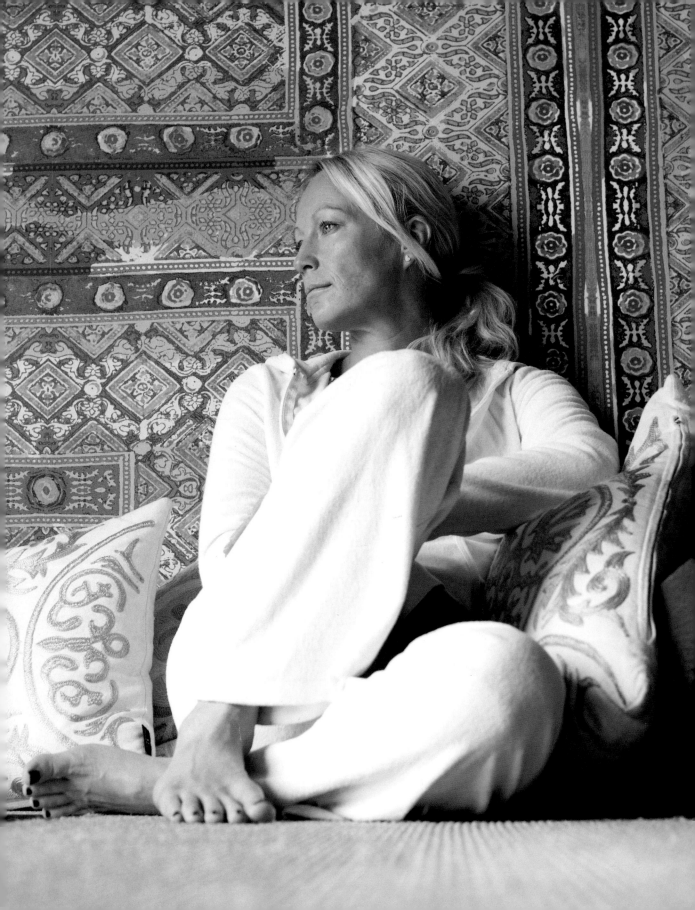

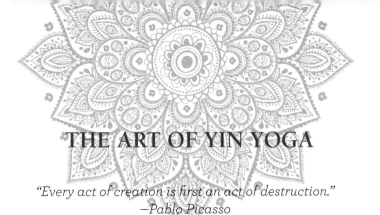

THE ART OF YIN YOGA

"Every act of creation is first an act of destruction."
—Pablo Picasso

If you think too much or not enough, you accumulate tension in your body and mind. If you work with your body or if you don't, you get tension. You get tension from sleeping too much or not at all. You even get tension from eating a heavy protein diet, a carbohydrate diet, or a vegetarian diet. Tensions appear in the different layers of the human personality. They arise in the our emotional, muscluar, and mental systems.

In yoga, we deal with aspects of tension through a wide-lens objective. We understand that if one part of a person is tense, other parts are too. If the mind is tense, so is the stomach, and if the stomach is tense, then the whole circulatory system is too. Therefore, yoga empasizes the importance of releasing tension. Inner tension can manifest in unhappy life chaos and disorder in the social life, as well as in aggression and warfare between cultures and nations. Yoga claims that peace can only be achieved from within. I would say this is accurate, since we have tried for thousands of years to achieve peace in the world through religion, law, police forces, armies, and governments, and it still eludes us. To create a more peaceful world, we need to learn how to relax and balance our bodies and minds.

Einstein was able to scientifially prove what the yogis found thousands of years ago—that energy cannot be destroyed, it can only be transformed. As yogis, energy is what we work with and what we wish to alter and redirect to improve our overall health from the inside out. When our health stabilizes and we are able to keep our balance better, we can make a larger impact on the world around us.

All the methods of yoga aim to release blocked energy and rechannel it so it flows more freely. When you take a yoga class, you become quite aware of these blockages through feeling resistance, stiffness, tension, and sometimes aches in the body. Interestingly enough, through the yogic breath and by aligning your body in a more balanced way, these blockages start to release and you will experience profound effects on physical, emotional, and energetic levels.

When energy releases from where it has been held through tension or longstanding patterns of behavior or belief, it can show itself in several ways during or after practice, including the following:

- Emotional release ("good" or "bad" emotions)
- Shakiness
- Lightheadedness
- Feeling "spacey"
- Muscular spasms or releases

These effects are all normal signs that tension is releasing. However, if some of these sensations are prolonged, they could be signaling another kind of problem, so it's a good idea to see a doctor or therapist to see if there is something more to it.

As I mentioned in the introduction, yogic philosophy states three different tensions:

1. *Muscular tension.* Relates to the body itself and to the nervous system and endocrinal imbalances. These are easily released through deep relaxation in body and mind. Yin Yoga, yoga nidra, and restorative yoga are all great techniques to do so.

2. *Emotional tension.* Stems from the dualities of our life such as hate/love, success/failure, happiness/sadness, and loss/profit. Emotional tension is difficult to ease and release since we often have a difficult time expressing our feelings and emotions freely. Yin Yoga is a great tool for relaxing the emotional structure of the mind.

3. *Mental tension.* Comes through excessive mental activity of any sort. Our conscious mind is constantly registering our experiences and collecting them. From time to time they explode on us and we react. Yin Yoga and meditation can help us to relax the nervous system and the brain so that we can release the subconscious mind.

Most of us spend nearly every waking moment connecting to the world around us, as experienced through our five physical senses of taste, touch, sight, smell, and hearing. As we grow up and move through life on this physical plane, we identify more with this physical mode of existence, defining ourselves by how we look, what we wear, where we go. But we are so much more than this.

Karma means "action." It is, in many ways, the essence of being alive. In Tantric philosophy, karma is why we come into being in the physical plane—to work out the seeds of action we carry within us.

There are two levels of karma: *universal karma* and *individual karma.* (We sometimes refer to these as the "big" karma and the "little" karma.) The universal karma is the progression of action, will, or maturation throughout the universe, which we are all a part of. For example, your individual actions contribute in some way, large or small, to the path of human history, and the path of human history affects your own individual life. The individual karma is your own path of action in this lifetime, in this corporeal body.

Viveka (clarity, discrimination) is the clear vision we must bring to our karma to see it for what it truly is. We achieve viveka in the samadhi state when we can experience ourselves and our existence without ego or judgment. Over time, we increase our ability to bring this clarity into our moment-by-moment living.

Karma is our reason for being. The "action" of karma is more than the actions you take in your life; it is also the action of your manifestation as a human being and even the manifestation of the universe from the Big Bang onward. Your karmic fingerprint is the seed of what makes you unique as an individual human being. In a very real sense, you are your karma.

SVADHYAYAD ISHTADEVATA SAMPRAYOGAH.
"Through self-study one ascertains one's necessary path to spiritual enlightenment.
Traditionally this path is represented by an individualized spiritual deity."
(Yoga Sutras of Patanjali: Book 2, Sutra 44)

ISHTA Yoga

The illusions, attachments, and habits of our daily lives and limited day-to-day awareness create blocks in our bodies that impede the free flow of prana and the working out of our karma. Through the interconnectedness of mind, body, and spirit, we can encounter, affect, and release these blockages by working on physical, mental, and energetic levels.[6]

Meditation in particular allows us to step away from the patterns and challenges of our karma and see our greater roles, feel our places in the universe, and return to daily life with that new perspective. The expansion of ease, awareness, and prana that results from yoga is an expansion of our ability to live and follow our karmic path with ease and grace.

The word *science* in ISHTA is key to an understanding of ISHTA yoga. Far from an esoteric or antiquated set of concepts, ISHTA encourages a direct and personal application of yogic principles in a way that is precise, individual, and unifies an understanding of both the timeless universal principles and the uniquely modern aspects of being a yogi in the twenty-first-century Western world.

Hindus traditionally assign *ishta devatas*, or particular gods, who look after them throughout their lives, based on the qualities those deities possess or represent and the needs of the individual. Similarly—though in a non-religious sense—ISHTA practitioners feel everyone who practices yoga benefits from an *ishta sadhana*, an individualized daily practice that enables them to best look after themselves.

So let's investigate this tradition of yoga a little more deeply. To see where ISHTA yoga has its aims and intentions, it is helpful at this point to look more closely at the three sister sciences and how they coincide with each other.

Hatha deals with the physical body and how to balance its strengths and weaknesses to enable energy and awareness to flow freely; *Tantra* focuses on understanding the energetic body and its ability to bridge the physical and spiritual worlds; *Ayurveda* aims to understand the individual constitution of a person and how it affects his or her practice. All three pillars are equally important in the practice of ISHTA.

---

6   ISHTA Yoga Teachers' Training Manuals.

Hatha yoga is the science of strengthening the weaknesses in an individual and removing the stress and blockages that form in our systems through the practice of asana and pranayama. The balance between strength and weakness, effort and surrender, is *ha-tha* (sun-moon) yoga. It is interesting to note that the asana element is what most Westerners consider to be synonymous with Hatha yoga; however, asana is the basis of reestablishing harmony in the physical body so that you may breathe deeply and freely to practice and explore pranayama, the art of breathing.

Tantra embraces all aspects of our being, fulfilling that which Hatha yoga sets the stage for. Beginning with pranayama, it uses the mental, physical, and subtle bodies to establish yoga in your system, sometimes working with all three bodies simultaneously and in other cases individually. To exist in the state of Tantra is to reside in the fullest potential in every aspect of our being—and more, to understand that all these aspects are interrelated.

Tantra comes from the root words *tanoti*, expansion, and *trayati*, liberation. *Tantra* is the belief that our essential nature is divine, perfect "as it is," part of the universal consciousness, and filled with bliss. The practice of Tantra is the practice of expanding our awareness into this blissful state of liberation through awareness of our innate perfection and acceptance of ourselves and everything around us.

The tools of Tantra in practice are: pranayama, Kriya yoga, visualization, and all aspects of meditation. These yogic tools of Tantra must be combined with an understanding of the Tattvas. The Tattvas are the seed forces of our senses and of the five elements (space, air, fire, water, and earth), which are all that truly exists on this material plane of consciousness. Ayurveda means the science of life, the essence of what makes you alive. It is the study of prana, the vital force of life, and how it manifests uniquely in every individual.

In **Ayurveda**, these distinct forces are called the *doshas* and are given names: *Vata*, *Pitta*, and *Kapha*. The *doshas* are another system or expression of the five elements, built upon relationships to particular elements.

- *Vata* (air and space) is the force that motivates all movement and breath, even on a cellular level; it moves the cells of our bodies and the thoughts that move through the mind. Light and creativity are essential Vata characteristics.
- *Pitta* (fire and water) is the heat in our bodies, our metabolisms, our physical magnetism, and the power for metabolism in thought (thought, too, is a chemical

process). The digestive fire in our system is created by acid, which is the combination of fire and water; the fire of Pitta results in clarity and strength of thought.

- *Kapha* (earth and water) is the force that binds water and earth together and creates the flesh body. Steadiness, patience, and groundedness are Kapha qualities.

How the life force mixes with the elements and exists in every human being is unique; each human being has their own unique makeup of the doshas to suit their spirit and karmic tendencies. That unique mixture is called the prakriti, which is the constitution of a particular human being, or the constitutional makeup of the doshas in that human being.

The effect of our prakriti in the circumstances of our daily living creates our vrikriti, which is the state or condition our life force is in. In other words, our prakriti is the underlying immutable fingerprint and our vrikriti is the mutable, ever-changing result of the interplay of this prakriti with our living conditions, affected by stress, joy, injuries, illness, and the challenges and changes of daily life.

If our current circumstances and daily life do not "fit" us—if our vrikriti does not match our prakriti—this imbalance will create disharmony and disease on all levels of our being: mental, emotional, physical, and spiritual. Therefore, we first need a good understanding of our inherent nature (prakriti), and then an awareness of our vrikriti, so that through our yoga practice we can address the imbalances of our living to bring us into perfect balance and perfect health.

It is through this process—through the tools of Hatha, Tantra, and Ayurveda—that ISHTA yoga helps us to understand and address the unique construction and the unique needs of each individual.

The ISHTA Practice

Based on the above keystones, the ISHTA practice integrates the physical and energetic tools of yoga. Asana, pranayama, and meditation combine into a seamless practice that leads the individual to self-awareness, inner and outer equilibrium, and self-transformation. Believing that the Tantric state of liberation, bliss, and acceptance is our natural state, and the return to this state is the intent of the yoga practice, an ISHTA practice brings together asana to stretch, strengthen, balance, and release the physical body; pranayama and visualization to still and quiet the mind; and meditation to expand our awareness to the universal state of bliss.

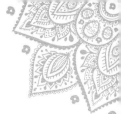

"Energy and consciousness become free. This is what ISHTA is about."
—Alan Finger[7]

Yin Yoga ISHTA Style

An ISHTA Yin Yoga class brings together asanas, pranayama, and meditation with the goal of releasing energy and liberating consciousness.

ISHTA Yin Yoga includes:

1. Energetic alignment through kriyas—focusing on the subtle body
2. Individual form—finding the appropriate pose to target the fascial area of interest
3. Freedom to use props to support the practice
4. Meditation

1. ENERGETIC ALIGNMENT THROUGH KRIYAS

ISHTA alignment begins with the Tantric principle that the physical body is the vehicle for our subtle bodies and all that goes with it—the mind, spirit, karma, and habits we carry with us. Thus, attention to the physical body always carries with it the awareness that physical movement directly affects these more subtle elements.

Next is the awareness that the physical and subtle bodies are intricately linked in ways that Western science is only beginning to understand and appreciate, and thus true alignment of the physical body *is* alignment of the subtle body, including the meridians, chakras, and nadi systems.

The balancing of energy and spirit through this marriage of physical and subtle is connected by the breath, which is the carrier of prana.

Finally, we remember that the original intent of physical alignment through the practice of asana was no more nor less than the ability to sit peacefully in meditation, where energy flows freely, the body is strong, quiet, and comfortable, and we come to yoga in the union of mind and body, breath, self, and universe.

---

7   ISHTA Yoga Teachers' Training Manuals.

This union of breath, body, and spirit enables us to experience ease, freedom, and joy in the bodies we live in on this plane, and to reconnect with the divine carried within that body.[8]

ISHTA alignment is:
- that which allows free and even breath
- focused on increasing the free flow of prana through the physical and subtle bodies
- alignment from the inside out, not just the outside in
- personalized to the individual's range of motion, strength, flexibility, and mental and emotional states
- safe for the physical body and healing for the mind and spirit
- that which creates space, balance, and freedom in the joints, the breath, the mind, and the spirit

As we learn in studying the subtle body, a human organism is a complex holistic system, a *yoga* of mind, body, and spirit. What's more, our internal state (in the form of the mind, spirit, and energetic body) and external form (in the form of the physical body) comprise an intimate and ever-evolving relationship, each affecting the other.

Our beings function best when we are in a state of *homeostasis*, or balance, not only within ourselves, but with the universe as well. As such, any physical movement or action ripples throughout our entire systems. Physical asana practice does not merely change the body; it changes the flow of prana, the movement of breath, the state of the mind.

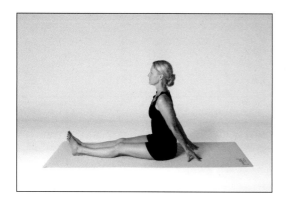

Correct pelvic alignment

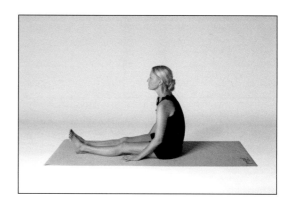

Incorrect pelvic alignment

---

8   ISHTA Yoga Teachers Manual.

In ISHTA Yin Yoga, we don't want to fall out of alignment, nor emphasise an active engagement of the muscular tissue to hold the body up. What we wish to do is create a natural alignment focusing on the skeletal strucure of the body. This is especially important in seated forward postures where the discs in the lower back and neck easily get compressed to an unhealthy limit. To avoid this, we advocate a slight active tilt in the pelvis.

To get to a better pelvic alignment, I advise sitting against a wall or on a folded blanket to elevate the pelvis or place blankets under the knees if they are sensitive.

"You can be in a room twenty years, trying to get out through the walls, the ceiling, the floor. It is when you finally discover the door that you find your way out. That's how it is with the soul. The average devotee may struggle his whole life trying to escape the bodily limitations by unscientific means, and by the paths only of devotion or discrimination. By Kriya Yoga, however, if he is sincere, he can escape quickly. Kriya Yoga takes one to spirit by the universal highway: the spine."

—Paramahansa Yogananda[9]

AROHAN AWAROHAN KRIYA

Kriya uses breath to alter energy patterns in the body, with active concentration on purifying the consciousness and the energy paths.

The most traditional forms of kriya practice involve simple breath awareness with repetition of mantras and visualization of energy patterns in the spine and central nadis of the subtle body. ISHTA yoga expands this definition to include further Tantric techniques, which utilize the mind to purify the physical and subtle bodies. All techniques combine the tools of breath awareness, subtle body attention, and mantra and visualization into powerful tools for directing and liberating prana. Kriya works from fascia. Asana works from muscles.

The Figure 8 kriya originates and terminates at the perineal body (root) at the pubic bone. Inhalation moves from the root, up the front of the body, crossing over at the jugular notch back to bindu (back of head), to brahmaranda (top of the head) , and into ajna (in the

---

9   ibid.

middle of brain). Exhalation moves from ajna to C7 (the cervical vertebrae in the base of the back neck), down the back passage of the body and back to the root (tailbone).

It is important to remember that the patterns followed in Arohan Awarohan are pre-existing breath and prana passageways in the fascia, nadis, and subtle points of the body. By visualizing Arohan Awarohan, you are purifying these pathways via the directing of your consciousness.

Arohan Awarohan is a very valuable practice for a number of reasons:

· Induces pratyahara (inner observing) by drawing the student's focus to the inner pathways of the breath
· Balances rajas and tamas gunas by balancing the front and back passages of the breath
· Opens flow in brahma nadi (central channel in spinal cord), bringing consciousness to its pure state

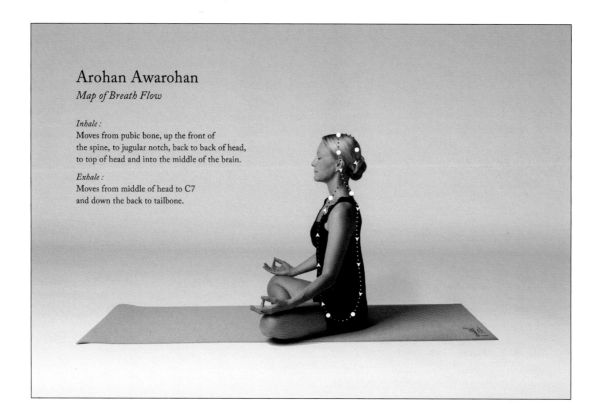

Arohan Awarohan
Map of Breath Flow

Inhale:
Moves from pubic bone, up the front of the spine, to jugular notch, back to back of head, to top of head and into the middle of the brain.

Exhale:
Moves from middle of head to C7 and down the back to tailbone.

INDIVIDUAL FORM—FIND THE APPROPRIATE POSE TO TARGET THE FASCIAL AREA OF INTEREST

To find the appropriate form to suit your body, we work with a focus on finding a fascial connection in a specific targeted area of the body. The targeted areas follow the different planes the spine moves in; flexion, extention, lateral flexion, and rotation. When one knows the targeted area one can find the appropriate pose that does not create compression, pain, or discomfort, but rather the connection with tension and sensation. The focus in ISHTA yin can also be different tensions. Sometimes, we do not want to find the physical tension, and instead just focus on the mental or the emotional tension. Then taking an easier pose— one that doesn't involve much physical challenge—might be more effective.

These poses are explained in chapter 6.

THE USE OF PROPS TO SUPPORT THE PRACTICE

Since ISHTA yoga has a more individual focus, one needs to accomodate the practice and find the appropriate adaptation in the poses at different times. As in any yoga, one needs to honor the present moment and how it affects us. So we always offer props like bolsters (round stuffed pillows), blankets, blocks, and mats to create a more individually adapted yoga practice that can aid the practitioner in avoiding misalignment due to tension. In all the seated poses, it is of great importance to try to avoid compression in the lower back. You can either place the fingers behind you and press them into the floor to create some length in the spine and remove unhealthy compression of the vertebraes, or you can put blankets underneath the sitbones, and maybe under the knees, to better support your posture.

PROPS.
- Yoga mat for good support
- Yoga blocks are good stabilizers
- Yoga blanket—the best Yin Yoga prop. To sit on and to create more relief or support.
- Yoga bolster for reducing pressure

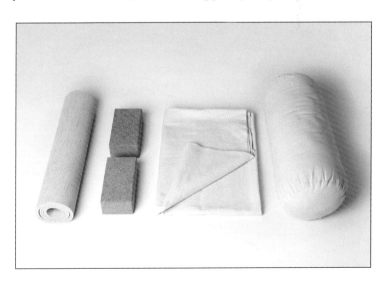

The Goal is Meditation

In ISHTA Yin Yoga, we work toward ending the practice with a short while of meditation. Try to gradually work up the minutes from 2 toward 6 minutes.

A. A nice way to move into meditation is to first find a comfortable seat, either with the help of props or sitting against a wall.

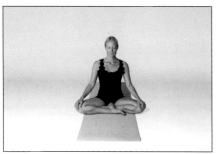 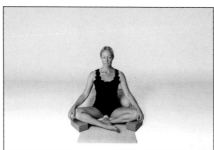 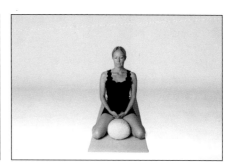

B. Then a couple of rounds of the breathing technique called *The Pendulum:*

1. Place your hands on your knees with the palms facing up.
2. Exhale and close the palms and make soft fists.
3. Open the right hand and inhale through the right side: at the end of the exhale, hold the breath and pause, closing the right hand into a fist again.
4. Open the left hand and exhale out the left side. Pause, hold the breath, and inhale through the left side with the left palm open.
5. Pause and close both hands. Then open the right palm and exhale out.
6. This is one round. Repeat this flow 2–6 rounds

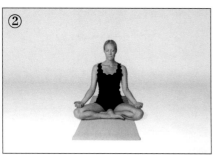 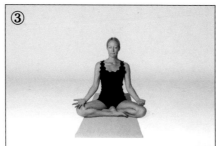 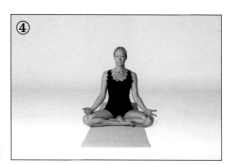

C. Once you notice that your mind's quiet and the breath softens, then start applying the Figure 8 kriya/ Arohan Awarohan, until your mind stills even more.

D. Then try to keep your attention on either a point in the middle of the chest/heart or at a point in the middle of the brain. And remain here for 2–18 minutes. You could put a timer on for the time you wish to invest in stillness.

E. When you have met your time, start breathing gently and bring the awareness back to the middle of the brain. Then bring your breath and awareness to you heart, then the navel, and lastly to the base of the pelvis.

F. Then come into Savasana. Aim for at least 5 minutes here.

G. Gently roll over to the right side (left side if pregnant to reduce pressure on Vena Cava[10]) and come up to sitting.

Place your right hand into a soft fist, placing it just at the pubic bone, shielding it with your left hand. Bow forward slightly and close your eyes. Center back and then place the palms together in front of the chest and thank yourself for your practice by saying *Namaste*.

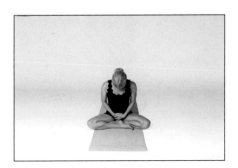 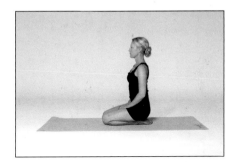

---

10   Vena Cava is the large vein that carries de-oxygenated blood from the lower half of the body into the right atrium of the heart.

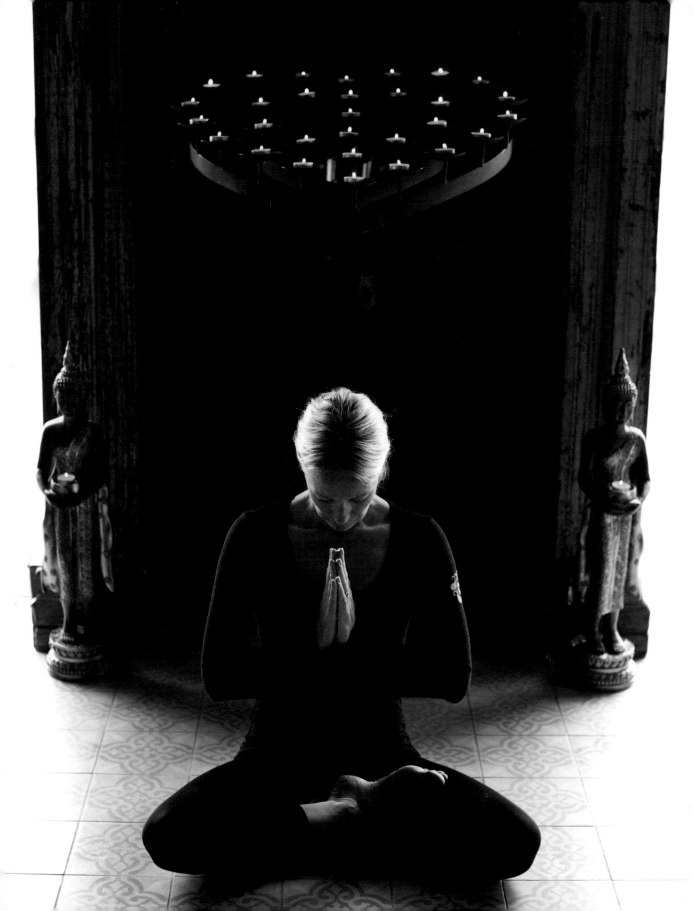

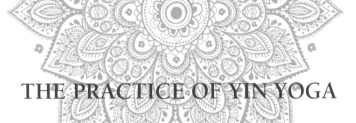

THE PRACTICE OF YIN YOGA

"Hearing Nada (centrally aroused sound), the mind (like a cobra), immediately forgetting everything and getting composed, does not run hither and thither."
—Hatha yoga Pradipika 4.97

As yogis, we ought to focus on techniques that help to create inner calmness and a settled mind. In the text *Hatha yoga Pradipika*, this is described as being bound by the bonds of *Nada* (the sound of our inner self; our Atman). The mind, having abandoned all fickleness, stands perfectly still like a lake with no ripples.

Yin Yoga is the art of yielding, recieving, slowing down, and relaxing into wonderment on an everyday basis. Your yoga practice should be guiding you to what you *need* to balance yourself rather than merely what you *want*.

The practice of Yin Yoga can help us come to that understanding of what is good for us as unique individuals. Through this, we can cultivate an active attention toward life that is not just about understanding what is happening to us, but rather becoming conscious of how we relate to what is happening to us.

The Principles of Yin Yoga Practice

Before we get into the yin asanas, let's take a look at Yin Yoga technique.

FINDING YOUR EDGE

When you come into a position, move slowly and gently into shape. Don't try to follow a picture or an idea of how far you should go in the exercise. In yoga there are no aesthetic ideals and no end results to strive for. Pause frequently and listen to your body. Wait for the body and mind to respond before going deeper into the position. Finding your limit doesn't always need to mean pushing yourself.

Many yoga practitioners lose their sensitivity to the body's signals as they go through the motions of a yoga practice day after day, perhaps focusing too much on achieving a physical goal, such as a sculpted body or mastering a new pose. Look instead for just the right amount of intensity in each exercise. Aim for a sensation that you, through the breath, can just *be* with during each moment of breathing, not having to *do* or fix anything.

BE STILL

At first, you will want to find movement in each position—you'll feel anxious, antsy, uncomfortable holding a single pose for an extended period of time. Try to resist the impulse to move around in each position. When you start to feel anxious, practice discerning whether those signals are coming from your body or from your mind. It's likely that the mind is telling you to hurry up and do something, just as the body is beginning to reap the benefits of relaxing into the pose.

A stressed or very active mind will tell you that your hair is out of place, or there's an itch that needs to be scratched. See if you can resist the urge to react to these distractions. Instead, imagine yourself releasing into the shape you're creating with your body. This will help to relax the muscles around the connective tissue each pose is trying to reach.

Movement can create stress on the connective tissue, which can lead to injuries. Move into a pose until you just begin to feel a "point of contact," a stretching sensation that tells you you're approaching your edge. Then allow the props or the surrounding muscles to support you as you become still. You will naturally sink deeper into the stretch as your body is ready. A good way to think about it is 99 percent stability and stillness, 1 percent challenge and contact.

STAY A WHILE

One recommendation is to hold the positions between one and three minutes for beginners and up to five minutes for more advanced practitioners. If you like, you can use a stopwatch to monitor the time. Use each pose to practice staying in the moment. Rather than giving up when you begin to feel anxious, see if you can experience the stillness as being valuable in itself, an opportunity to breathe evenly and freely and connect with your body.

MOVE WITH SOFTNESS AND RESPECT

Yin Yoga places you in positions that are challenging for joints, ligaments, and muscles; positions that can hurt you if you leave them too quickly or aggressively. When you come out of a position, do it *very* slowly and use your hands to support your legs, gently contracting the muscles you've just been releasing while in the pose. It's also beneficial to add a countermovement. For example, if you have been bending forward, sit upright and stretch backward gently.

In Yin Yoga, you challenge deep tissues that the body normally protects from getting stretched since they're easily damaged by force. You may experience some discomfort, some shaking, or a slight feeling of instability. This is normal, especially when you are new to the practice. However, if a position causes severe pain or makes you so uncomfortable that it affects your focus or breathing, then you've gone too far and need to slowly come out of the pose.

Other warning signs that you've pushed too far are feelings of extreme weakness or instability, muscle spasms, or misalignments that you can't correct. If you experience these things, take a break to breathe and then, if it feels right to your body, begin again, slowly and very carefully, stopping when you begin to meet your edge. Props may be helpful.

MINDFULNESS AS A BASIC THEME

Mindfulness is something we always come back to. It is the backbone of Yin Yoga. Consciously and with friendly curiosity, examine the experience of this moment.

When and Where to Practice Yin Yoga

One really great aspect of Yin Yoga is that you can receive a lot of benefits from a short practice of even fifteen minutes, and you can do it pretty much anywhere. For physical benefits only, you can do the poses even while talking on the phone.

Since Yin Yoga deliberately targets the deeper connective tissues, we need the muscles to be cool and relaxed. If the muscles are warm and active, they will tend to absorb most of the tension of the stretch.

When to pratice Yin Yoga depends on what you would like to achieve through the practice. Some options:

- When your muscles are cool
- Before an active yang practice (before the muscles become too warmed up)
- Early in the morning (when muscles are cool)
- Late at night (to calm down before sleep)
- In spring or summer or in hot climates (to balance the hot, yang weather)
- When life is very hectic (to balance more yang energies in our life)
- After travelling (flying, driving, etc., tends to increase yang)
- During menstruation (yin is good to restore and conserve energies)

So when we are moving through hectic times in life, a gentle Yin Yoga practice can be very beneficial. However, Yin Yoga is not recommended if you are feeling lethargic. If you have been sitting at a desk for eight hours in the middle of winter, a more active practice is a much better choice.

A yin practice is very portable. You can bring it with you wherever you go. You don't need to be at a yoga studio, unless you want to be inspired and taught by a great Yin Yoga teacher, and you do not even need a yoga mat or exercise clothes. We don't want to sweat, but to create greater circulation so we feel an inner warmth that doesn't come from sweating, but rather from contentment.

Yin Poses
There are not nearly as many asanas required in the yin style of yoga as are found in the more active practices. There are about three dozen postures at most, excluding variations.

The yin areas of the body generally targeted in the practice are between the knees and navel, the lower body. Since the poses are held longer, you can fit fewer into a typical session, compared to the yang styles of yoga where one pose may be held for as few as five breaths.

Paul Grilley lists eighteen poses in his book *Yin Yoga,* along with some more active yang poses to be used between the yin poses to counterbalance. He states that the more yin quality your practice has, the less variety is needed, so the emphasis is placed on a few basic postures.

Following is an overview of some of the poses I recommend to start with. There is an image showing the nature of the pose, but keep in mind that how you look in a pose is not important. Instead, focus on the sensation and the connection to the area the pose targets. The connection could be physical, mental, or emotional.

I list some benefits of each pose as well as things to be aware of, such as contraindications, and how to modify poses to work best for you and your body.

Keep in mind that not all poses are right for everybody, so be gentle and respect your boundaries and limitations. Do not worry much if the pose you are trying doesn't work for you; there are many other ways to target the same tissues. Look at the options suggested to find the pose that works better for you.

Many of the following asanas might look very familiar to you, and you might say, "Oh, I know this pose, I have done it before." But you will notice that the name of those poses are different in Yin Yoga. The pose looks the same but the intention is different. The yin pose of the Butterfly is identical to its yang version, Baddha Konasana, if you just look at the picture. However, in Baddha Konasana, we target and engage the muscles and stretch them. In the yin practice, we relax muscles and aim the intention into our joints and deep tissues. We are aiming for just being with the connection to the area, not moving through it. You want to be alert and pay attention in the pose rather than running away from the connection with the experience.

THE MOST COMMON YIN YOGA POSES AND THEIR TARGETED AREAS

TARGET AREAS
In Yin Yoga, it is of value to work with a Target Area, a specific muscular/fascia area, since you then can find the appropriate pose of modification in order to connect better to the fascia in that specific area.

Some common target areas are: Quadriceps (front thighs), Psoas (hip flexor), Quadratus Lumborum (Lumbar spine), Hamstrings (back of thighs), Erector Spinae (spine muscles), Adductors (inside of thighs), Abductors (outside of thighs), piriformis (back of pelvis), Gluteus muscles (attached to back of pelvis), abdominals (front of spine, core), shoulder girdle, and upper thoracic spine (area in between the shoulder blades).

Different poses can target the same area, but since our form is unique, we might find the connection to the area through different poses. And this may change from day to day or it might be the same for life.

When you come into the pose, listen to your body and notice if you feel a sensation (just the beginning of a sensation, very soft) at the targeted area. If not, try one of the other positions that might work better for your body. You do not want to feel pain or be very uncomfortable nor have that sense of the mind getting more restless just entering the pose. If you feel okay and have sensation but only mental discomfort remains, the kriya and the breath will help you settle. Also, the use of props as needed is a great help to move into a state where you have connection to the targeted area but you have enough mental space so you can close your eyes and move inward and focus deeper on the breath and the visualization.

The targeted area is there to serve you as a way to find the connection with the fascia in that area. And the kriya is of use for you to move from the external, inward and then deeper into conciousness.

OUTLINE OF POSES
Anahatasana
Ankle stretch
Bananasana
Butterfly
Half butterfly
Cat pulling its tail
Caterpillar
Child's pose
Dragon
Frog/Deep child's pose
Happy baby
Half happy baby
Reclining twist
Shoelace
Snail
Supta padangusthasana
Sphinx/Seal
Square
Squat
Dragonfly
Swan
Sleeping swan
Viparita Karani
Savasana

ANAHATASANA

This pose focuses on stretching the upper and middle back, opens the shoulders, and softens the heart. The targeted areas are Erector Spinae, Trapezius, shoulder girdle, and the diaphragm. This pose can be used as a gentle warmup to deeper backbends and it is nice to do this pose after a series of lower backbends.

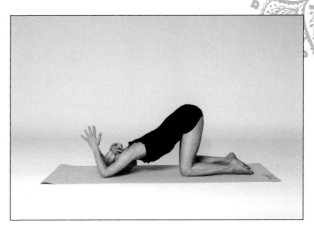

GETTING INTO THE POSE
Start on your hands and knees, walk your hands forward, allowing your chest to drop toward the floor. Keep your hips right above your knees and point the sitbones back, trying not to compress the lower back. If possible, keep your hands shoulder-width apart. You do want to avoid a "hanging" sensation in the shoulders.

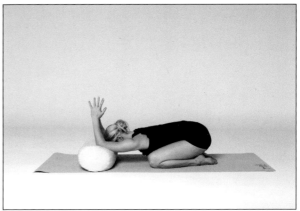

ALTERNATIVES AND OPTIONS
- If you experience shoulder pain or strong tingling in your fingers or hands when lifting your arms overhead, move them farther apart or put a bolster under your belly alongside the spine, or underneath the elbows. If the tingling does not stop, do Child's Pose instead.
- If knees are uncomfortable here, place a blanket underneath them.
- You can do this pose with just one arm forward at a time, resting the head upon the other forearm.

COMING OUT OF THE POSE
Start first by connecting to your breath and then either move back into Child's Pose or slide forward onto your belly.

CONTRAINDICATIONS
- If you have a neck injury be especially gentle as this asana could strain it further.
- If you feel pinching in the back of the shoulders, you may be reaching a compression point. Moving the arms farther apart may release this.

COUNTERPOSES

I usually advise to gently move into Child's Pose because it is a mild forward fold. Then carrying on with some cat-cow sequences usually feels nice.

RECOMMENDED HOLD TIMES
Three to five minutes

ANKLE STRETCH

This pose opens and strengthens the ankles and it is a great counterpose for squatting or toe exercises.

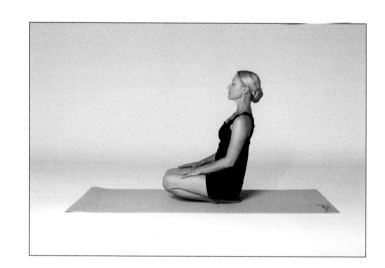

GETTING INTO THE POSE
Begin by sitting on your heels. If your ankles or knees complain, this may not be the pose for you. Then, you can try and slide a blanket or bolster under the knees to reduce the pressure on the ankles and feet.

COMING OUT OF THE POSE
Lean forward and bring your hands to the floor beside the knees. Slowly lift one foot at a time, circling the foot around its own joint. Then step one foot at a time back to a Downward-facing dog.

CONTRAINDICATIONS
- If there is any sharp pain in the ankles, try placing a blanket or towel under the feet to cushion them or do not do the pose.
- Knee issues may prevent you from sitting on your heels. Placing a rolled-up towel behind the knees may be very therapeutic, or a cushion can be used between the thighs and calves.

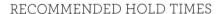

RECOMMENDED HOLD TIMES
About one minute. This is a relatively intense pose that shouldn't be held for a long time if there is a lot of discomfort.

OTHER NOTES
This is a nice counterpose for many postures that stress the feet, such as Toe Squat, Regular Squat, and sitting meditations.

BANANASANA

This is a wonderful way to stretch the whole side of the body. It works the spine in a lateral flexion (side bend) from the iliotibial (IT) band to the tops of the side ribcage. You stretch the oblique stomach muscles and the side intercostal muscles between the ribs.

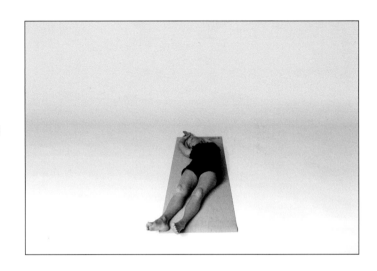

Lying on your back with your legs together and straight on the floor, reach the arms overhead and clasp your hands or elbows together. With your buttocks firmly glued to the earth, move your feet and upper body to the right. Arch like a nice, ripe banana. Be careful not to twist or roll your hips off the floor. When you feel resistance, pause.

When your body opens more, move both feet farther to the right and pull your upper body farther to the right, as well. Again, pause at the place where you begin to feel resistance and patiently explore that before going further. Dont forget to do both sides.

COMING OUT OF THE POSE
Simply straighten your legs and bring your arms down. Then gently hug the knees into the chest.

CONTRAINDICATIONS
• If you experience tingling in the hands when extending your arms overhead, you may need to place a folded blanket under the arms or keep the hands on the belly.

- If you have lower-back issues, move into pose cautiously and avoid going too deeply. You could put a bolster underneath the knees.

RECOMMENDED HOLD TIMES
This can be held for three to five minutes.

Butterfly/Half Butterfly

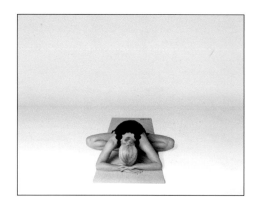

Here you stretch the lower back without requiring loose hamstrings. If the legs are straighter and the feet are farther away from the groin, the hamstrings (back of thighs) will get more of a stretch. If the feet are in closer to the groin, the adductor muscles (inside of thighs) get stretched more.

GETTING INTO THE POSE
Sit on a folded blanket, then bring the soles of your feet together and then slide them away from you. Allowing your back to round, fold forward, lightly resting your hands on your feet or on the floor in front of you.

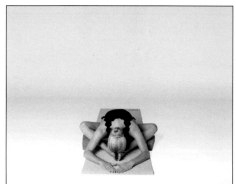

ALTERNATIVES AND OPTIONS
- If the neck is tight or stressed, support the head in your hands or on a bolster, or slide blocks under the thighs.
- If the back doesn't like this pose, you can try to do half butterfly; take one leg at a time, or do this pose toward a wall in the reclining variation—lie down, keeping legs in butterfly, leaning against the wall.

COMING OUT OF THE POSE
- Use your hands to *slowly* roll up.
- Before straightening your legs, lean back on your hands to release the hips, then slowly straighten each leg.

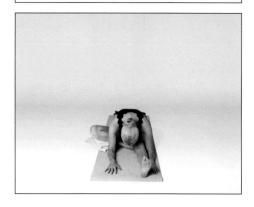

CONTRAINDICATIONS
- If you have sciatica, elevate the hips by sitting on a cushion, until the knees are below the hips, or avoid this pose entirely. Beware of hips rotating backward while seated; we want them to rotate forward.
- If you have any lower back disorders that do not allow flexion of the spine, then do not allow the spine to round; keep the back as straight as you can or do the reclining version.
- Avoid dropping the head down if the neck has suffered whiplash or has reverse curvature. Use a bolster to support your head.

COUNTERPOSES
- Sit up, or do a gentle sitting backbend
- Lie on stomach, which is also a gentle backbend
- Gently sit up and move the upper body side to side or do a gentle twist.

RECOMMENDED HOLD TIMES
Three to five minutes

OTHER NOTES
Many students will automatically go into a tight butterfly, because of their yang training. Feel encouraged to move the feet away, forming a diamond shape with the legs. This pose can be nice for pregnant women because the legs are separated, providing space for the belly.

CAT PULLING ITS TAIL

This is a nice counterpose to strong forward bends (such as the Snail or Caterpillar) and a great alternative to Dragon. It mildly compresses the lower back and it opens the quadriceps and upper thighs.

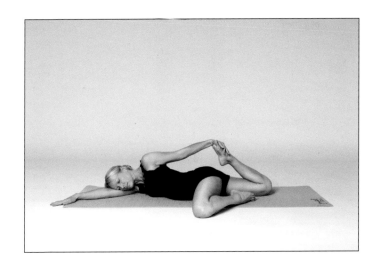

GETTING INTO THE POSE
Start by lying on your right side, reclining on your right elbow. Keeping your bottom (right) leg straight, bring your top (left) leg

forward and to the side. Bend the right leg, bringing that heel toward your buttock. Reach back with your top (left) hand and grab the bottom foot. Pull the foot away from you.

From here, come to your belly. Then roll onto your left side. Keeping your bottom (left) leg straight, bring your top (right) leg to the side. Bend the bottom leg, bringing that heel toward your buttock. Reach back with your top (right) hand and grab the bottom foot. Pull the foot away from you.

ALTERNATIVES AND OPTIONS

The more challenging version is to recline and straighten the top leg and look over your shoulder to the bottom foot. This version becomes a reclining twist with a backbend. For a softer approach, lay on a bolster. This makes a good alternative to Dragon for those sensing pinching in the groin or hip.

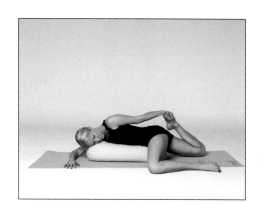

COMING OUT OF THE POSE

Gently release the bottom foot and roll onto your stomach. Straighten the bottom leg and roll onto your back.

CONTRAINDICATIONS

If you have lower back issues, move into the pose very gently. You may not be able to pull the foot away at all. Try using a bolster.

COUNTERPOSES

Sometimes it feels nice to do a gentle cat-cow stretch or roll over onto your back and hug the knees to the chest to release the lower back in a gentle forward fold. A Child's Pose also feels nice after this pose.

RECOMMENDED HOLD TIMES

- Can hold for three to five minutes as a reclining twist
- One minute if done as a counterpose to a forward bend

CATERPILLAR

This pose stretches the ligaments along the back of the spine and compresses the stomach organs, which helps strengthen the organs of digestion.

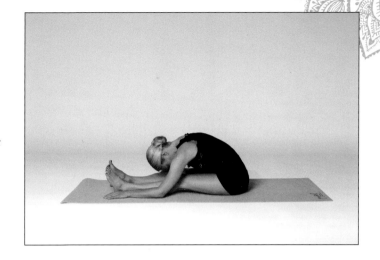

GETTING INTO THE POSE
Start sitting on a cushion or a folded blanket with both legs straight out in front of you (you can also keep a folded blanket under your knees). Make sure you have a pelvic forward tilt in your pelvis before gently folding forward.

ALTERNATIVES AND OPTIONS
*   If your hamstrings are really tight, you won't be able to fold forward enough to allow gravity to draw you down. Bend your knees and place a bolster underneath; allow the back to round fully. If that doesn't work, sit up on more cushions.
*   If your neck feels strained by the weight of the head, support your head on a bolster.
*   You can do this pose with the legs up a wall, which is called viparita karani (see later in chapter). This variation is great for those with SI-joint issues or if pregnant.
*   If knees feel strained, keep a small bend in the knees and a folded blanket underneath the knees.

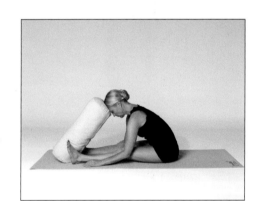

COMING OUT OF THE POSE
*   Gently start to yield back into a neutral, central position.
*   Once you are up, lean back on your hands to release the hips and then shake out the legs.

CONTRAINDICATIONS
*   If you have sciatica, elevate the hips by sitting on a cushion, until the knees are below the hips, or avoid this pose entirely.

- If you have any lower back disorders that do not allow flexion of the spine, do not allow the spine to round—keep the back as straight as you can.
- If the hamstrings are very tight, the knees should be bent and supported by a bolster, allowing the spine to round.

COUNTERPOSES
- Sit up or do a gentle sitting backbend
- A seated twist

RECOMMENDED HOLD TIMES
Three to five minutes

OTHER NOTES
- Keep muscles relaxed, especially in the legs.
- Make sure the tops of the hips are tilted forward. If the hips are rotating backward, sit on higher cushions and bend the knees more. Fold forward enough that gravity is doing the work, not your muscles. If you are not folding forward, you won't be able to relax completely. Let gravity have you. Yin is all about surrendering.

CHILD'S POSE

GETTING INTO THE POSE
Sit on your heels, allowing the belly and chest to round forward onto the thighs. Let the forehead rest toward or on the floor. In the extended variation, you should extend the arms forward along the floor and let the palms face down. Close the eyes.

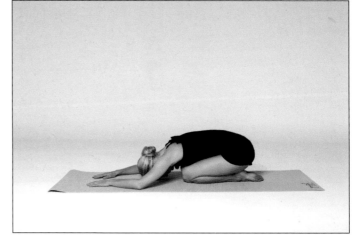

This pose is a great tension release for the pelvis and lumbar spine as well as a calming pose, where one can start ones practice. Also, it is easier to sense Arohan and Awarohan in this pose than some other poses.

COMING OUT OF THE POSE
To Adho Mukha Svanasana: With arms extended forward, press the palms into the floor and lift through the elbows. Come forward onto all fours and curl the toes into the mat.

Press down through the hands and heels and lift the hips back and up.

OPTION
- Support the lower back by resting on a bolster. This also puts less pressure on the knees.
- If the knees, shoulders, or neck are too sensitive, another option is to do apanasana, hugging the knees, resting on the back.

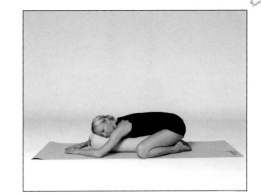

COUNTER POSES
- A gentle cat-cow sequence
- Downward-Facing dog

RECOMMENDED HOLD TIMES:
Three to six minutes

DRAGON

This is a deep hip and groin opener that gets right into the joint and stretches the back leg's hip flexors and quadriceps—and it has many variations to help work deeply into hip socket.

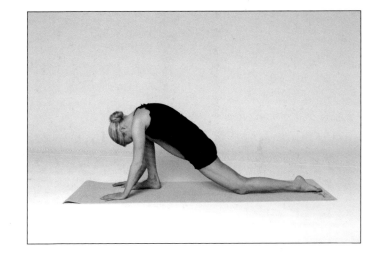

GETTING INTO THE POSE
Begin either on hands and knees or in Downward-Facing Dog. Step one foot between the hands. Walk the front foot forward until the knee is right above the heel. Slide the back knee backward until you sense a gentle connection with the hip flexor area. You do not want too strong of a connection. Keep the hands on either side of the front foot.

ALTERNATIVES AND OPTIONS

If the back knee is uncomfortable, place a blanket under it, rest the shin on a bolster, or tuck the toes under and lift the leg off the floor.

ALTERNATIVE DRAGONS

- The first alternative pose is a simple, low lunge called Baby Dragon. If you like, you can rest your hands on blocks.
- A deeper option is to place both arms on the front thigh. For more depth, come down on the elbows or rest them on a bolster or block.
- In the lower image, one hand pushes the front knee to the side, while the chest rotates to the sky.
- Another option is to instead take *Cat Pulling Its Tail*.

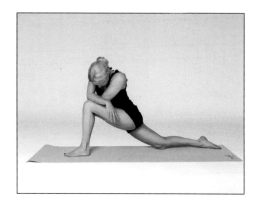

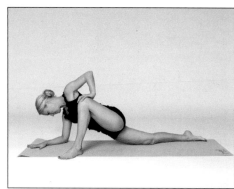

COMING OUT OF THE POSE

Move gently to Downward-Facing Dog position, *very* slowly.

CONTRAINDICATIONS

Can be uncomfortable for the kneecap or ankle. Support the back knee with a blanket, or place a bolster under the shin, allowing the back knee to be off the floor.

COUNTERPOSES

- A short Downward-Facing Dog is fantastic. Bend one knee, lifting that heel and pushing the opposite heel down, and then switch sides repeatedly.
- Child's Pose followed by cat-cow feels really good after Downward-Facing Dog and before switching to the other side of the Dragon.

RECOMMENDED HOLD TIMES

Hold for three to five minutes.

FROG/DEEP CHILD'S POSE

This is a deep groin opener (especially the adductors; inside of thighs) and it also provides a slight backbend, which compresses the lower back.

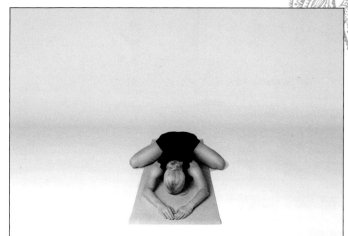

GETTING INTO THE POSE
Start in Child's Pose and slide both hands forward, separate the knees, but remain sitting on the heels. This is also known as the Wide-legged Child's Pose.

ALTERNATIVES AND OPTIONS
- Extend one arm at a time, which is safer than extending both arms forward. The other arm can be bent with the head resting on the forearm.
- Allow the hips to come forward if the pressure in groin or hips is too severe.
- Alternately, keep toes together and allow hips to go backwards.
- You may rest the chest on bolster, to relax upper body.
- If the shoulders are uncomfortable, spread the hands wider apart.

COMING OUT OF THE POSE
Either sit back into Child's Pose or slide forward onto your belly, bringing your legs together.

CONTRAINDICATIONS
- If you have a bad back, use classical Child's Pose.
- Knees can be uncomfortable, so use padding under the knees. Or do this pose on your back with feet wide, in the so-called Happy Baby.
- If the neck is stiff, rest the forehead, not the chin, on the floor or on a bolster.
- If prone to tingling in the hands when you extend the arms overhead, you may need to move the hands wider apart or closer together. If that doesn't help, do one arm at a time.

COUNTERPOSES
- Child's Pose
- Cat-cow
- Lie on the back, hug knees to chest, and rock side to side, or move knees in circles.

RECOMMENDED HOLD TIMES
Three to five minutes

Happy baby/Half happy baby

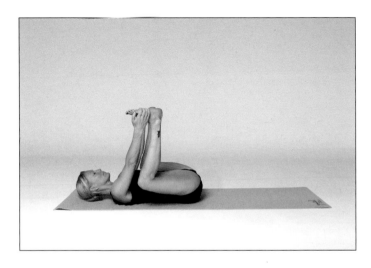

Here is a deep hip opener and one that can use arm strength, rather than letting gravity do the work. This pose helps with releasing and decompressing the sacroiliac (SI) joints.

GETTING INTO THE POSE
Start lying on your back, hug the knees to your chest. Grab the soles of the feet, the ankles, or the back of the legs. Open the feet so that they are above your knees, and pull the knees toward the floor alongside your chest. Relax your head and shoulders down to the floor.

ALTERNATIVES AND OPTIONS
- Half Happy Baby (like an upside-down Baby Dragon), holding one foot at a time.
- If you're very tight, you may use a belt to hold your feet, or you may do this against a wall. It is like a lying down Squat.
- You can hold on to the back of the thighs or onto your feet in a version that is more like reclining Butterfly.
- Keep the tailbone low to the ground.

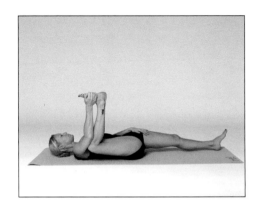

COMING OUT OF THE POSE
Slowly release the feet, placing them on the floor, with the knees bent. Pause for a moment. Hug the knees and rock softly from side to side.

CONTRAINDICATIONS
This can become a mild inversion: you may want to avoid this posture if you have your period or if you have very high blood pressure.

COUNTERPOSES
- Gentle cat-cow sequence
- Hug the knees

RECOMMENDED HOLD TIMES
Two minutes if you are actively pulling with the arms, but if you relax the arms you can linger up to five minutes.

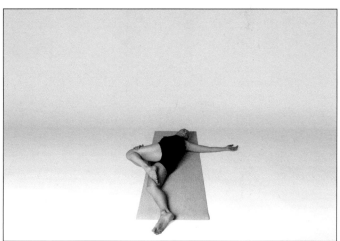

RECLINING TWIST

Twisting at the end of the practice helps to restore equilibrium in the nervous system and release tension in the spine.

GETTING INTO THE POSE
Lying on your back, draw both knees into your chest. Open your arms to the side like wings and drop the knees to one side.

ALTERNATIVES AND OPTIONS
- Place the lower foot on the thigh of the top leg to get a deeper opening sensation in the lumbar.
- If the shoulder is still floating, place a blanket under the shoulder or a bolster along the spine.
- Experiment with turning your head to either side and notice how the sensations change.

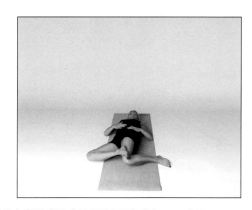

COMING OUT OF THE POSE
- Slowly roll onto your back and hug the knees into the chest to release the sacrum and lumbar.

COUNTERPOSES
- Hug the knees and rock on your back from side to side

RECOMMENDED HOLD TIME
Three to five minutes

OTHER NOTES
- An excellent final pose of the practice
- You can slide right from this pose into Savasana.
- It is important not to push the rotation here. Relax. Let gravity do the work.

Saddle

This pose provides a deep opening in the sacral-lumbar arch and it also stretches the hip flexors and quadriceps. If the feet are beside the hips, this becomes a good internal rotation of the hip.

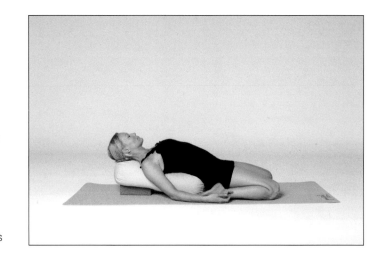

GETTING INTO THE POSE
Start with simply sitting on the heels and notice how this feels. If there's pain in the knees, skip this one. If your ankles are complaining, try a blanket under them or skip the pose—try Happy Baby instead. Lean back on your hands, creating a little arch to the lower back. Check in with how this feels. If you can go further, come down onto your elbows.

ALTERNATIVES AND OPTIONS
- A blanket or rolled up towel under the ankles can relieve pressure there.
- Lift the hips even higher by placing a block between the feet and under the buttocks.
- If this is too deep for the lower back, do the Sphinx pose.

- You can sit on a bolster to reduce pressure on knees and lower back. Or lay back on the bolster.
- You can also stretch just one leg at a time for reclining Half Saddle. Sit on the edge of a bolster with one leg bent back and one leg in front with the foot on the floor (as shown) and lay down gently on the bolster. Make sure the lower back can rest comfortably on the bolster. You can sit upright here if the sensation is immediate in the front thigh. If you can only go as far back as your elbows, rest on a bolster to relax here. There are various ways you may use bolsters—stack two crossways under the shoulders, use just one, or place one lengthwise under the spine.

COMING OUT OF THE POSE
- If you can, come back up the way you went down, propping yourself up on your elbows and then onto the hands. Lie down on your belly, straightening your legs slowly to allow the knees to release.
- Support yourself on your hands.

CONTRAINDICATIONS
- If you have a bad back or tight sacroiliac (SI) joints, be cautious or avoid pose altogether.
- Knees can be tested too much here.
- Ankles can protest.
- If you experience any sharp or burning pain here, you must come out.

COUNTERPOSES
- Child's Pose: move into it slowly. You may need to rest your head on your palms before coming into a full Child's Pose.

RECOMMENDED HOLD TIMES
One to five minutes

SHOELACE

This is a great hip opener, and when performed as a forward fold, it helps decompress the lower spine.

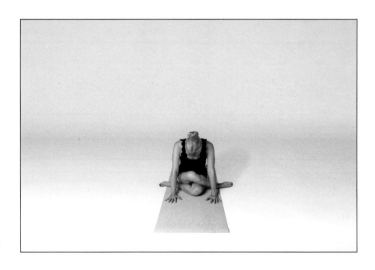

GETTING INTO THE POSE

There are several options for coming into this pose. One way is to begin by kneeling on all fours then placing one knee behind the other and sitting back between the heels. A second approach is to begin by sitting on your heels and then slide onto one buttock and bring the outside foot over toward the opposite hip. A third approach is to begin by sitting cross-legged and then draw one foot under the opposite thigh and the other foot over toward the opposite hip. Try not to sit on the feet but rather slide them as far forward as they can go. Anchor both sitting bones to the ground. You want to feel a sensation that targets the outside of the hip/pelvis. There should be no pain in sacrum, knees, or lower back. If that happens, do not do the pose and try another option.

ALTERNATIVES AND OPTIONS

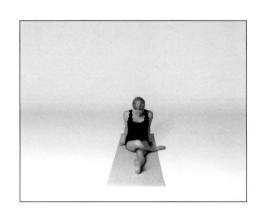

- If hips are tight, sit on a folded blanket to tilt them forward. Make sure you tilt the pelvis forward and don't tilt the spine in the lower back.
- For those with SI-joint and knee instabilities, try this pose reclining.
- If the bottom knee complains, do the pose with the bottom leg straight. If the top knee complains, place a bolster or blanket under that knee. If this is still too hard, sit cross-legged and fold forward.
- When folding forward, you can support the head with the hands, leaning the elbows onto the thighs or a block or a bolster.
- If sensations are too intense in the hips or knees, remain upright or take more weight into the hands and arms.
- You can add a side bend/lateral flexion or a twist here.

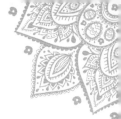

COMING OUT OF THE POSE
Lean back to release the hips and slowly straighten the legs.

CONTRAINDICATIONS
- This pose can be hard on the pelvis and knees and can aggravate sciatica. If you have sciatica, elevate the hips by sitting on a cushion so the knees are below them. Beware of hips rotating backward while seated; we want them to tilt forward.
- Pregnant women should not fold forward after the first trimester. Do the option lying down instead.

COUNTERPOSES
- Lean back and stretch the spine.
- Downward-facing dog

RECOMMENDED HOLD TIMES
Three to five minutes per side. So if you add a twist you could do three minutes the neutral way, then two minutes with a side bend right side, two minutes a side bend on the left side, and gently back to neutral.

OTHER NOTES
- It is nice to follow this with Sleeping Swan before doing the other side or do a seated twist afterward to counterpose.
- Keep weight on the sitting bones when you come forward, preventing the weight from moving into the knees.

SNAIL

This pose is one of the deepest
releases of the whole spine and it
relaxes the heart and brings more
blood flow to the head, drains the
lungs, and compresses the internal
organs, giving them a great massage
through the pressure the pose gives.

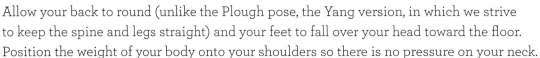

GETTING INTO THE POSE
Start lying on your back. Lift your
hips and support them with your hands.
Allow your back to round (unlike the Plough pose, the Yang version, in which we strive
to keep the spine and legs straight) and your feet to fall over your head toward the floor.
Position the weight of your body onto your shoulders so there is no pressure on your neck.

ALTERNATIVES AND OPTIONS
*   Support the back with the palms, a folded blanket, or a bolster.
*   There are many intermediate stages to this pose. For beginners, or those not wishing
    to invert, replace this pose with a seated, straight-leg, forward fold like the Caterpillar
    or Viparita karani with legs up the wall pose (also a great option for pregnancy and for
    women through their period).
*   A nice alternative is Happy Baby, which allows the sacrum to lift off the floor. Allow the
    spine to fully round. Do not try to keep the spine straight and the hips high.

COMING OUT OF THE POSE
*   A simple way to come out is to keep the knees bent and hold your hips. Allow yourself
    to slowly roll down. Your head will likely lift up as you come down. Don't strain to keep
    your head on the floor.

CONTRAINDICATIONS
*   Avoid if you have any neck problems since this pose puts pressure on the neck.
*   Not recommended for anyone with high blood pressure, upper-body infection, vertigo,
    glaucoma, or a cold; also women who are pregnant or who are experiencing their
    menstrual cycle may find it better not to do this pose.

- If you have any lower back disorders that do not allow flexion of the spine, then do not attempt this posture.

COUNTERPOSES
- When you come out of this pose, lie down for a few breaths with the knees bent and feet flat on the floor and breathe into your belly.
- Child's Pose

RECOMMENDED HOLD TIMES
Three to five minutes

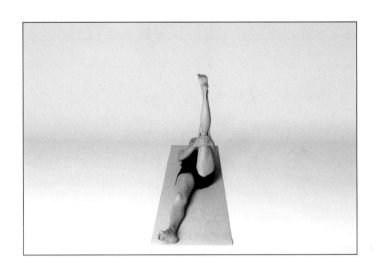

SUPTA PADANGUSTHASANA

GETTING INTO THE POSE
From a supine position, bring one knee into the belly. Keep the spine in neutral on the floor. Straighten the leg and grasp behind the thigh with both hands or bring a strap around the ball of the foot and draw the hands down the strap until the shoulders return to neutral. Soften the legs and relax the feet. Bring the drishti (gaze) to your hands or toes.

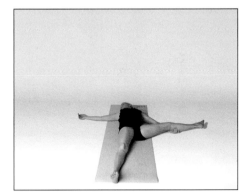

This pose targets the back of the thigh and leg and the sacrum. After a couple of minutes, fold one leg over the other as shown, keeping the two sides of the pelvis directly over each other.

Variation: Keep the spine in neutral and the resting leg pressing into the ground. Externally rotate the raised leg and open the leg to the side.

COMING OUT OF THE POSE
Softly draw the knee back down into the belly. Release the leg to the floor.

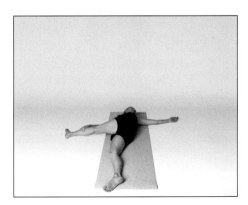

Variation: Stay grounded through the pelvis and resting leg as you internally rotate the raised leg back to center. Bring the knee into the belly and release the leg to the floor.

ALTERNATIVES /CONTRAINDICATION:
- For those with SI-joint instabilities, take care and do not do the version where you reach the leg outwards. Rotate the spine so that the hips are stacked on top of each other to target the rotation in the Thoracic spine.
- If you have a herniated disc in the spine, just perform the first variation, and leave the rotation out.
- A nice alternative is viparita karani, legs up the wall pose.

Sphinx/Seal

These two poses are the backbends of Yin Yoga. They stimulate the sacral-lumbar arch, which tones the spine. People with bulging or herniated disks may find this very therapeutic. In the full Seal pose, the stomach may receive a lovely stretch, as well.

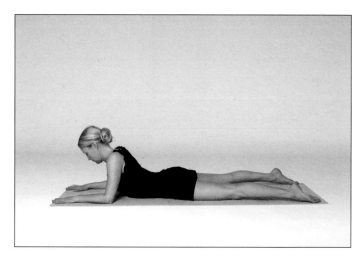

GETTING INTO THE POSE
Lie down on your belly. Come up on your elbows and move the elbows just in front of your shoulders, propping yourself up. Relax your buttocks and legs. Notice how this feels in your lower back. If the sensations are too strong, move your elbows further ahead, lowering your chest closer to the floor. If you like, you can place your palms flat on the floor in front of you like a Sphinx.

ALTERNATIVES AND OPTIONS
- For a gentle Sphinx, rest on the ribs, sliding the elbows away to reduce compression in the lower back. Simply lying on your stomach may be enough of a backbend for you.

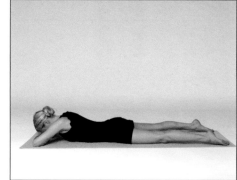

- Alternatively, you can place a bolster under the upper belly and relax completely.
- Seal pose with straight, locked arms is the deepest pose; let the hands rotate outward a little. Slide your hands away to lessen the intensity.
- You may spread the legs apart to deepen the sensations in the lower back.
- You may prefer to keep the legs together to release the sacrum or to spread the sensations more evenly along the spine.
- You can place a bolster or blanket under the pubic bone or thighs to soften the pressure.
- To support your neck, try resting your head in your hands or your chin on your fists.

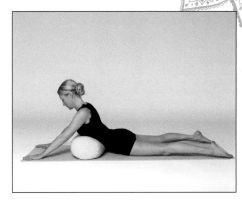

COMING OUT OF THE POSE
- To come out, slowly lower your chest to the floor. Turn your head to one side and rest your cheek on your palms. You may wish to decompress the lower back more by sliding one knee up.

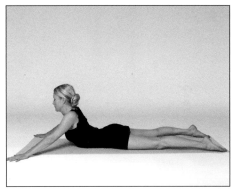

CONTRAINDICATIONS
- If you have a bad back or tight sacrum, try laying on your stomach with a blanket under your pelvis and see if that feels okay. Just breathe in the belly.
- If there are any sharp pains here, do NOT do this pose.
- Avoid this if you're pregnant unless you can consult with an experienced teacher that can give you professional advice and variations.
- Avoid if you have a headache.

COUNTERPOSES
- Child's Pose is a nice, gentle, forward fold. However, move into it slowly. You may need to rest your head on your palms.
- Cat-Cow

RECOMMENDED HOLD TIMES
- Sphinx can be held longer than Seal
- For Seal, start with one-minute holds, then lower down, rest, and repeat several times
- up to five minutes

OTHER NOTES
Ideal for adding breathfocus and Arohan/Awarohan practice.

Square

This pose is quite tricky to get into. Listen to your body and honor its restrictions. The targeted area is the outer hips/buttocks/IT-band and you should not feel any pain in knees. This is a deep opening of the hips through strong external rotation and it decompresses the lower back when folding forward.

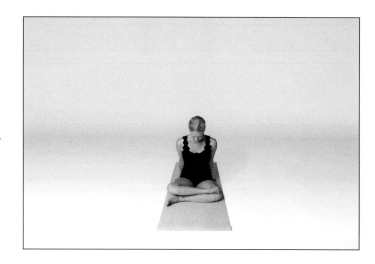

GETTING INTO THE POSE
For a gentle start, come to a cross-legged seat. Move your feet forward until your shins are parallel to the front edge of your mat (it is often called the firelog pose). Gradually move toward keeping feet and knees parallel each other. Flex the feet to protect the knees.

ALTERNATIVES AND OPTIONS
- Folding forward stretches the lower back and can intensify the stretch in the hips. If you can't come forward, sit on a cushion.
- If you experience tightness or discomfort in the knees, or if the knees are high off the floor, you can place blankets or some form of support under the knees.

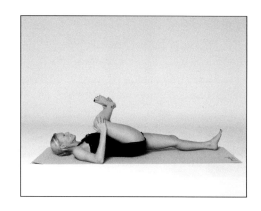

- You can do a variation where one leg is extended forward and the foot of the bent leg is under the knee of the extended leg.
- Another variation is to do this pose on one leg only and reclining.
- Other alternatives include Shoelace or Swan.

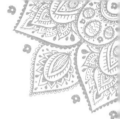

COMING OUT OF THE POSE
Lean back and slowly straighten the legs out in front of you.

CONTRAINDICATIONS
- Watch the pressure on the knees; if the hips are too elevated, the pressure will go there.
- Can aggravate sciatica. If you have sciatica, elevate the hips by sitting on a cushion until the knees are below the hips, or avoid this pose entirely. Beware of hips rotating backward while seated; we want them to rotate forward.
- If you have any lower back disorders that do not allow flexion of the spine, then do not allow the spine to round; keep the back as straight as you can.

COUNTERPOSES
- Sit with hands on the floor and stretch the spine into a gentle backbend.
- Bounce out the legs and tighten/release the knees a few times.

RECOMMENDED HOLD TIME
Three to five minutes per side

OTHER NOTES
- If you're a beginner, you may tend to bring your feet close to the groin. Make sure this isn't simply a cross-legged sitting posture; we want to feel this in the outside hips.
- If you already feel sensation simply sitting, then cross-legged is stressing the hips a lot and that is your version of Square pose.

SQUAT

This pose works toward greater openness in the hips and inner thighs. It releases tension in the lower back and strengthens the ankles.

GETTING INTO THE POSE
Start by standing with the feet hip-width apart. Squat down and bring your arms in front of you, hands in prayer position and elbows pulling lightly against the knees or shins or lean the head into your hands.

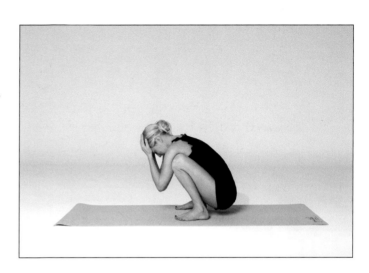

ALTERNATIVES AND OPTIONS

- If your heels are off the floor, use a folded blanket or bolster under them. We want the body to relax. Another option if the heels are off the floor is to widen the distance between the feet.
- Knees and feet should point in the same direction. If they are not, spread the feet wider or rest the heels on a folded blanket or on a bolster.
- If you experience great tension in the neck and shoulder, lean the head toward a bolster.

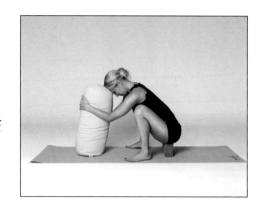

COMING OUT OF THE POSE

- An easy exit is to just sit down and then slowly straighten the legs out in front of you.
- A more challenging exit is to come to Dangling by straightening the legs and folding forward. As you straighten the legs, align the feet so that they are pointing in the same direction as your knees.

CONTRAINDICATIONS

- If hips are too tight, this pose can torque the knees; if you have a knee imbalance, avoid this pose. A better option is to lay on your back and hug your legs.

COUNTERPOSES

- Dangling pose—standing forward bend, helps to release accumulated tension in the knees and back afterward
- Ankle stretch

RECOMMENDED HOLD TIMES

Two to three minutes at one time. This is a nice pose to revisit a couple of times during the practice.

OTHER NOTES

- A recommended sequence is to go from Dangling to Squat, back to Dangling, back to Squat, again and again, holding each position for one to two minutes.

DRAGONFLY

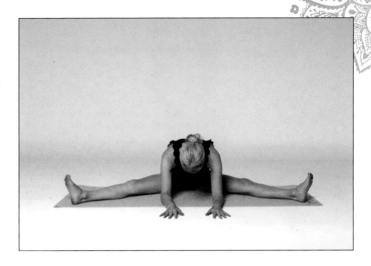

This pose focuses on the inner thighs, groin, and the back of thighs. It provides a gentle opening to inner knees, though you shouldn't get a straining sensation in the knees. If you do, don't widen the legs so much.

GETTING INTO THE POSE

Come into a seated position with a folded blanket under your seat (and sometimes under your knees, too, if you have sensitivities in your knees). From there, gently spread your legs wide apart. This pose requires a forward tilt in the pelvis. If a cushion or blanket doesn't give that, then sit against a wall to help you with that alignment. Use the hands as a support behind you or walk the hands gently forward in front of you. You want to have a soft roundness in the spine, but not slouch forward. Relax your legs and feet.

COMING OUT OF THE POSE

- Use you hands to hold the pose while you gently come out of the pose. Do it at half the speed of what you believe is slow.
- Once your spine is erect, it is nice to lean back on your hands to release the hips, tighten the leg muscles, and drag or lift your legs to bring them together. Softly bounce or shake out the legs.

ALTERNATIVES AND OPTIONS

- You can use a bolster to raise the hips. Then place two rolled blankets underneath the knees to protect from overstretching the knee joints.
- You can keep hands behind the back or rest elbows on a bolster.
- If the knees feel bothered, tighten the quadriceps to close the knee joint, or bring legs closer together.
- If the hamstrings (back of thighs) feel too tight, bend the knee(s) and place a bolster under the thigh(s).
- It is quite nice to use a bolster under the chest if you are close to the floor.

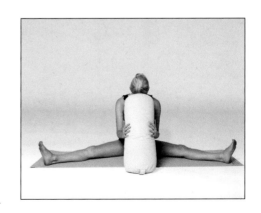

THE PRACTICE OF YIN YOGA   97

- Tension in the neck or shoulders can be minimized by supporting your head in your hands or leaning your forehead onto a standing bolster.
- You can move into a sitting-up twist or lean to the side into a lateral flexion. If you do this, then hold it for two minutes and very gently come back to neutral before peforming the same action on the opposite side.

CONTRAINDICATIONS

- This pose can aggravate sciatica. If so, then elevate the hips.
- It is important that your hips do not tilt backwards while seated; we want them to tilt forward.
- If you have any lower-back disorders that do not allow flexion of the spine, then do not allow the spine to round; keep the back as straight as you can.

COUNTERPOSES
- A seated backbend is nice afterwards.

RECOMMENDED HOLD TIMES
Three to ten minutes

Swan/Sleeping Swan

The swan is a marvellous way to open up more range of motion and circulation in the hips, allowing gravity to do the work. You get a strong external rotation of front hip and it provides a soft stretch for the quadriceps (front thighs), hip flexors (front hip), and buttocks areas where we normally carry a lot of tension.

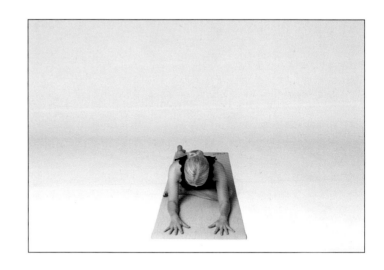

You can come into this pose from standing on all fours. Slide your right knee toward your right hand and lean a bit to the right, and check in with how your right knee feels. If there is no strain or pain, flex the right foot and move it forward. If the knee feels stressed, bring the foot closer to the right hip. Now, center the pelvis so you carry even weight on both sides. If the buttocks are off the floor, then slide a blanket under the hips. In Swan, you lean into your hands with your spine upright, whereas Sleeping Swan is more of a forward bend.

COMING OUT OF THE POSE
Use your hands to push the floor away and slowly come up. Tuck the back toes under, plant your hands in Downward-Facing Dog position and then on all fours for a couple of cat-cow stretches.

ALTERNATIVES AND OPTIONS
- If you experience pain or strain in the knee or groin, then do this pose lying down on your back instead to reduce the pressure on the hip and knee joint.
- To protect the front knee, keep the foot flexed before coming forward.
- Keep the weight back in the hips as you lower yourself.
- Stay on the hands with the arms straight, or come on to the elbows.
- You could lay on a bolster placed lengthwise under the chest.
- Other alternatives include Shoelace and Square Pose.

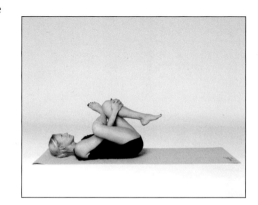

CONTRAINDICATIONS
- If you have sensitivities in the knees (especially any problems with the meniscus), watch the pressure and do the modified reclined version instead.
- If hips are very tight, the same advice with the reclined version applies well.

COUNTERPOSES
- A Downward-Facing Dog before Child's Pose
- Cat-cow stretches

RECOMMENDED HOLD TIMES
Three to four minutes on each side

Savasana

This pose offers time to release and relax. Rest is necessary for the body and mind to become stronger and healthier. Savasana allows all major muscles to relax and allows you to experience a neutral body without muscular effort and gives Relaxation response benefits.

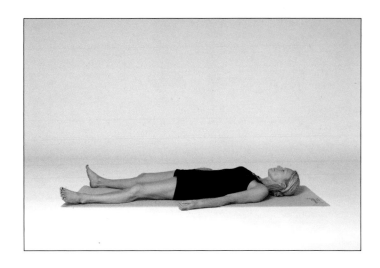

Savasana symbolizes the end of your practice—a natural completion to the journey you have been on. Savasana is a pose where you can practice attentiveness rather than falling asleep. See if you can start paying attention to the energies flowing inside you. This is an ideal time to develop your ability to feel your energies. It is difficult to do this when you are in the postures. Practicing watching the energies during your Savasana will assist you in feeling energy flowing at other times. At first you may have to pretend you can feel these energies. Pretending will help you look closely at these areas. In time, you will notice the energy flow more easily.

If you are practicing on your own, you may want to set a timer for your Savasana. For Yin Yoga, since the muscles were not used a great deal, making Savasana a shorter part of the practice is okay—maybe 5 percent or 8 percent of the practice time will suffice.

GETTING INTO THE POSE

From a seated position, bend the knees and place the feet on the floor. Roll down the spine, keeping the sides of the body as even and lengthened as possible. Extend the legs. Relax the shoulder blades onto the floor and allow the arms to rest comfortably away from the body. Let the legs fall open (generally they will come into a natural external rotation here). Close the eyes.

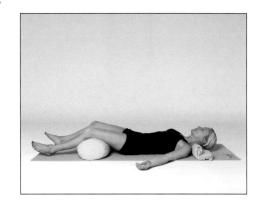

For a more supported variation, place a bolster under your knees, a blanket under your neck, and cover yourself up.

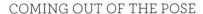

COMING OUT OF THE POSE
Bring attention back into the physical body by deepening the breath and rotating the joints or stretching gently. Draw the knees into the belly. Roll on to one side with the knees drawn in. Rest for several breaths. Keeping the head low and the neck released, press the hands into the floor and gently roll up the spine to come to a neutral seat.

CONTRAINDICATIONS
- Pregnancy: Lay on the left side with a bolster between the thighs.
- If you cannot lay supine (breathing difficulty, etc), try laying on the right side.

VIPARITA KARANI

This pose affects the Relaxation response, reduces fluid pressure in lower body, releases tension in the hamstrings and lower back, encourages full complete breathing, rebalances and redistributes lymph and hormonal flows, reduces overall blood pressure, and slightly increases blood flow to head.

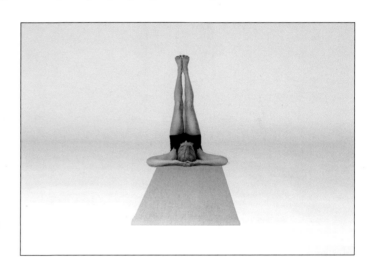

COMING INTO THE POSE
Sit with one hip against the wall, facing sideways, with knees bent and feet on the floor. Swing both legs up the wall, pivoting the torso down onto the floor and creating a 90 degree angle with the body where the wall meets the floor. Release the arms onto the floor, nestling the shoulder blades down into the floor and spread wide across the back.

Propped variation: Place blankets folded into small rectangles or squares under the sacrum and back of the head.

Arm variations: Hands rest on belly; arms extend out to the sides at shoulder height; or arms in "cactus" variation (deeper backbend/breath opener/shoulder release).

COMING OUT OF THE POSE

Note: All resting poses have a subtle but very strong impact on the body's fluid and energetic systems. Transitioning out of resting poses should always be done very slowly and gently.

Draw the knees down into the belly. Roll onto one side with the knees drawn in. Rest for several breaths. Keeping the head low and the neck released, press the hands into the floor and gently roll up the spine to come to a neutral seat.

MODIFICATIONS

- Leg variations on wall: Dragonfly or butterfly with a strap around legs
- Tight or injured hamstrings/lower back: Elevate calves on to seat of chair

CONTRAINDICATIONS

- Hamstring or back injury—chair variation
- Pregnancy and menstural cycle—elevate the torso with a bolster or pillows.
- Extreme high or low blood pressure—elevated torso variation as above
- Hiatal hernia and just operated your eyes—avoid this pose.

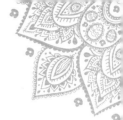

Yang Poses as Counterposes

CAT-COW SEQUENCE

PHYSICAL BENEFITS
- Releases muscles of the upper back, shoulders, and spinal extensors
- Strengthens muscles of the arms, shoulders, chest, and core

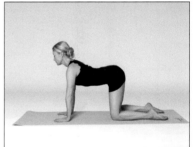

This is a great sequence to use between Yin Yoga holds to increase circulation in and around spine and to release any accumulated tension in the area.

Stand on all fours and align knees hip-width apart and stack them directly under the hip joints. Align wrists shoulder-width apart and stacked directly under the shoulders, or slightly forward. Ground the weight evenly through both knees and both palms, and evenly throughout each hand.

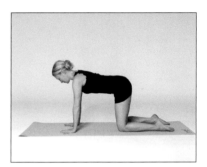

Cow: Inhale and curl the toes, press the hands down and gently stretch the chest and sternum forward (with the top of the shoulder blades moving toward each other) creating a forward arch in the upper back

Cat: Exhale and gently round the spine like a cat; the tailbone curls toward the floor and the spine rounds. Flatten the tops of the feet against the floor. Pressing down through the hands and feet, tip the pelvis back and draw the tailbone toward the floor. Draw the navel toward the spine and lift the back toward the ceiling.

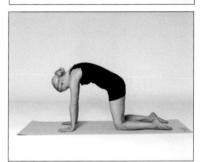

Repeat several times as needed for you to feel revived after a Yin Yoga held pose. Let the flow of the breath move you through this sequence. A nice variation is called the *Bear just out of Hibernation*, where you move freely, letting the movement take you to different areas around the spine, pelvis, and shoulders, pausing where there is a nice sensation.

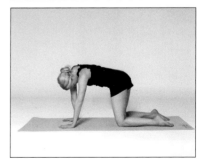

ADHO MUKHA SVANASANA- DOWNWARD-FACING DOG POSE

PHYSICAL BENEFITS

- Stretches hamstrings and lower back
- Shoulder opener
- Mild inversion: Can reduce blood pressure, soothe headaches, prepare for deeper inversions
- Good for scoliosis: Look at placement of hands, feet, hips, and shoulders to find balance and length through both sides of torso
- Creates space between the vertebra in the spine

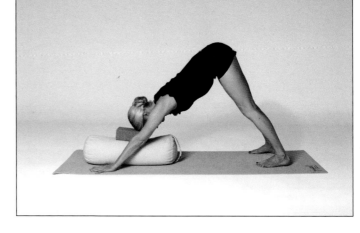

This pose is an ideal counterpose after a series of forward folds or gentle backbends. Just come into it and hold for a couple of breaths before you continue to the next Yin Yoga pose.

GETTING INTO THE POSE

Stand on all fours, spread the fingers comfortably wide and press down evenly into the hands, and press the toes into the floor. Keep pressing the hands into the mat as you lift the knees off the floor, bringing the thighs towards the belly. Extend the legs as much as you can while maintaining the length in the spine.

COMING OUT OF THE POSE

Release the knees to the floor.

Parsva Vajrasana—Mermaid

Physical Benefits

- Stretches muscles between the ribs, expands breath in side ribs
- Shoulder opener
- Builds stability in hips and pelvis
- Excellent for scoliosis

Contraindications:

- Shoulder injury
- Severe breathing challenges
- Rib injuries
- Knee injury

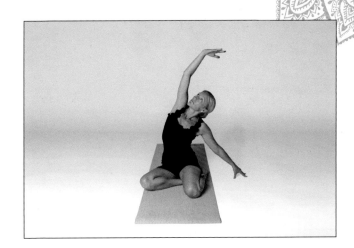

This is a nice side bending pose or gentle twist to use between seated poses like after a long forward bend to neutralize the spine and energy within.

GETTING INTO THE POSE

From sitting on the heels (Vajrasana): Sit over to one side of the feet, tucking the bottom toes over the top ankle. Walk the hand on the same side a few inches outside the shins, pressing down through the opposite hip. Extend the other arm up and over so that you are extending fully through the top side, from the hip pressing into the floor to the fingertips lengthening up and overhead. Rotate the ribcage open to the forward wall and lift the top side ribs toward the ceiling. Release the shoulder blades on to the back, deepening the arm bones into the shoulder girdle, and relax the shoulders away from the ears. Gaze to the top under the upper inner arm. Pause here and take a couple of deep breaths.

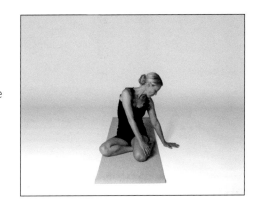

For a rotated version of this pose, gently rotate outward from center. Pause and extend the spine, breathe for a couple of breaths, and then softly return back to center.

COMING OUT OF THE POSE

To Vajrasana: Root into the sitbone of the extended arm side and contract the top-side waist to lift the torso back into neutral. Lower the top hand down alongside the body. Shift the hips into the center to sit on your heels. Repeat on the opposite side.

Shalabhasana—Locust Pose

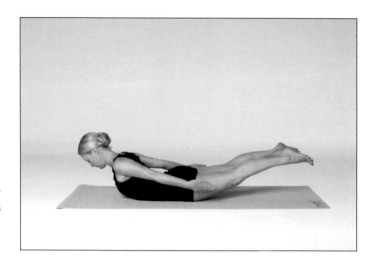

PHYSICAL BENEFITS
- Strengthens all major muscles of the back body: hamstrings, buttocks, spinal extensors, back of upper body, etc.
- Releases muscles of the chest, throat, and respiratory diaphragm
- Works while lengthening muscles of abdominal core
- Balances the muscles of the shoulder girdle
- Opens breath

CONTRAINDICATIONS:
- Cannot lie prone (pregnancy, some digestive issues)
- Spinal conditions: practice with caution

This pose can be integrated in the pre-Yin Yoga asana sequence or during the practice, after a series of forward folds. I recommend that you start by laying on the belly first for a couple of breaths. Just hold the pose for four to six breaths. Then return to Child's Pose before continuing on.

GETTING INTO THE POSE

From prone position (lying on the belly): With the hands by your sides, turn the palms to face the mat. Stretch back through the toes or press them into the mat; gently firm the thighs up toward the ceiling. Roll the shoulders back as you draw the chest forward and up and allow the arms and hands to lift in line with the chest.

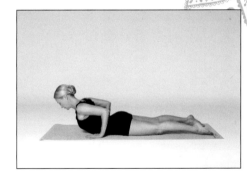

Press the front hip bones into the mat, keeping space in the lumbar region, and lengthen back and up through the legs as you draw the chest forward. Keep the centerline of the thighs, knees, and ankles facing the floor, the neck relaxed, and the jaw soft. Let the gaze rest on a point about 45 degrees forward along the floor.

COMING OUT OF THE POSE

To prone position: Keep the legs lengthening back as you lower the tops of the feet, the torso, chest, and head back down to the floor. Relax arms alongside the body. Rest the forehead on the floor or turn the head to one side.

SEATED TWIST

PHYSICAL BENEFITS

- Strengthens abdominals, spinal extensors, and rotator muscles of the spine
- Lengthens abductors/outside of legs
- Balances muscles of the shoulder girdle and chest

This is a nice counterpose after a seated forward fold. Come gently in and out of the pose and just remain for a breath or two while in the pose.

COMING INTO THE POSE

From a seated position, cross the right leg over the left, placing the right foot along the outside of the left thigh with toes facing forward.

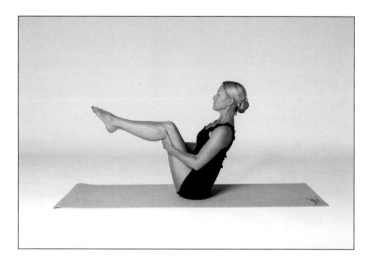

Full variation: Bend the left knee, drawing the foot back in line with the outside right hip.

Modified variation: Keep the left leg extended. Lift the ribcage up off the hip points and rotate toward the bent right knee, keeping the spine long and the center of the head, sternum, and belly in line above the center of the pelvis. Bring the right hand behind you and the left forearm or elbow to the outer right thigh. Gaze forward along the floor, approximately in line with the top hip. Repeat on the left.

COMING OUT OF THE POSE

To a seated position: Root down firmly through both sitbones and release the torso and head back to the center. Gently counter-rotate to the opposite side before coming back to center.

NAVASANA—BOAT POSE

PHYSICAL BENEFITS
- Strengthens all muscles of the core: abdominals, spine muscles, hip flexors
- Encourages smooth breathflow
- Aligns and balances joints and muscles of the shoulder girdle

Navasana is a good pre-asana Yin Yoga pose or for after a backbend series to counterbalance the pressure on the spine.

COMING INTO THE POSE

From seated: Bring the hands to the floor behind you. Bend knees with feet on the floor ahead of you. Press into your hands, lift through the core and the thoracic spine, and begin to unfold the shins parallel to the floor. Stay here, or lift off the hands, balancing on your sitbones, and extend the arms forward parallel to the floor. Stay here, or extend the legs straight, bringing them into a diagonal line, and elevate the palms toward the toes or overhead to the ceiling. Gaze to your palms or toes.

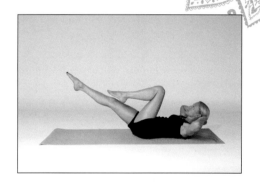

COMING OUT OF THE POSE

Press the sitbones and backs of the thighs firmly into the ground. Lift through the belly as you lead with the chest to bring the torso back to an upright position.

Special Circumstances

CONTRAINDICATIONS/CAUTION:

- All forms of damage to the spine should be taken very seriously, so be sure to honor your or your students' (if you are a teacher) physical health and know that yoga can not always solve everything. If you are weary or uncertain, always consult with an experienced and knowledgable yoga teacher (for modification or alternatives to accommodate and adapt to your condition), physician, or physical therapist before embarking on a practice.

- In Yin Yoga, I advise being conservative, meaning don't take any chances or go to the extreme in poses. Yin Yoga is not all about exploring the physical edges. It is more about coming to the first stage of an edge, just where you feel a connection to the area in mind for that pose. There is a big difference between pain and discomfort. Pain is NOT okay in yoga, but discomfort can totally be. Discomfort is a dynamic space for us to look into and use as a realm of inquiry around what drives us and creates tension. In this realm we will discover this, which is impossible if we move to the extreme edge and just use breath and other techniques "to survive and push through." Yin Yoga is not about that; rather, it's about exploring the surroundings in a sensation.

- Since we all will find different tensions in this practice and it will change from moment to moment, day to day, it is of great benefit to gradually cultivate a meditative state of mind (observing and yielding) during the poses to calm the nervous system and slowly move more to sattva guna: balance. Therefore, the implement of Arohan and Awarohan kriya in the practice when settled into the pose is of utmost benefit for a practitioner of Yin Yoga.

- Specific areas to be wary of: the joints, especially the neck, lower back/sacrum/SI-joint, and knees. Be open to modifying poses and also using support props. For those with any pelvis and spine imbalances, I recommend doing all the forward bends lying down and toward a wall.

- For those with knee injuries, be careful with poses like Saddle, Child's Pose, Swan, etc. that put too much strain on the knee, and choose other options like the modifications lying on the back.

- The meditative aspects of yoga are very favorable during pregnancy, but caution should be exercised because of the elevated levels of the hormone *relaxin* that works on softening of ligaments. Therefore, Yin Yoga for pregnant women ought to be more of a meditative, stress-reducing practice. Pregnancy is not a period during which we should push our physical limits. Provide support for thighs and knees during hip-opening exercises and avoid strong backbends (Sphinx/Seal. Do seated backbend leaning on hands behind the body and also gentle cat-cow) or rotations (better to do reclining twists, gently focusing on the breath). Also do not hold the poses for more than three minutes and make sure to move slowly (preferrably the *Bear just out of Hibernation* or *Adho Mukha Svanasana*) after the poses. Try to work on breathing, focus, and presence more than searching for bodily concessions.

- Make sure you always have the hips higher than the knees, which tilts the hips forward. This is to maintain the normal curvature of the spine in forward bends and to avoid hyperextension of individual segments of the lumbar spine, which may cause deterioration of the ligaments or irritation of the tissues.

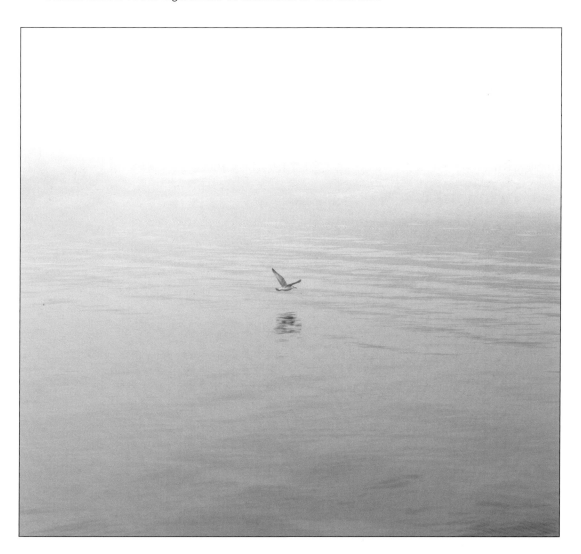

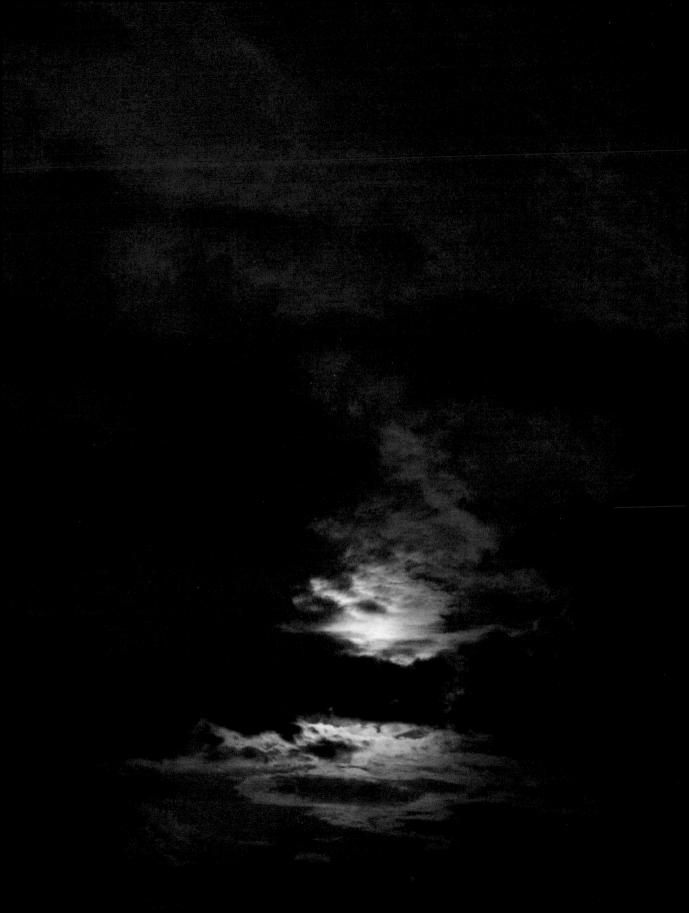

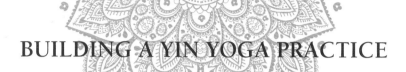

BUILDING A YIN YOGA PRACTICE

When one studies the goal of asana practice, one clearly sees that asana should help us reduce tension in the body and mind, strengthen the bodily tissues, increase circulation, and create close liaisons between the different polarities within. All this so the yogi can sit and meditate, which is the goal of yoga itself—the ability to attain a clear, attentive, and balanced mind.

So How Does One Get There?

Well, we can't get there through thinking, through apps, or through Google, neither can we get there through reading a book or just living our life.

If we are going to succeed in achieving more balanced health, there needs to be a *practice*, a time that we set aside daily. This is a time during which we align our body, mind, and spirit and get closer to ourselves. I often see my practice as updating all my inner programs, like when you are updating your computer, so they function better and can communicate more easily with each other, without friction or disturbances.

To feel comfortable with sitting in meditation, we need to have a practice that works towards good alignment. All seated meditation postures aim for one thing: holding the back upright without slouching or strain so that energy can run up and down the spine more freely. The fundamental core of the meditation posture is the proper tilt of the sacrum and pelvis. This alignment is what you want for seated meditation. The placement of the upper body takes care of itself if the pelvis is properly adjusted. A good foundation in your yoga practice should include forward bends, hip openers, backbends, and rotations.

Some of the most known forward bends in Yin Yoga are those that combine forward bends and hip openers, such as the Butterfly, Half-Butterfly, Half-Frog, Dragonfly, and Snail. All gentle forward bending puts positive stress on the ligaments around the back of the spine and the lumbar spine and helps to prevent undue compression of spinal disks. The forward bends are performed with legs stretched forward, gently stressing the fascia and muscles around the back of the legs.

The Snail focuses on the entire back of the body, but with the target area focused on the upper spine and neck. The poses Butterfly, Half-Butterfly, Half-Frog, and Dragonfly stretch not only your back but also the fascia that crosses the sacro-iliac region.

The Shoelace and the Square both target the tensor fascie latae, the thick bands of connective tissue that run up the outside of the thighs. The Sleeping Swan stretches all tissues that otherwise prevent the external rotation of the thigh bone you need to sit with your legs crossed.

To balance these forward flexing poses, it is recommended to follow them with positions such as Sphinx/Seal, Dragon (hip-flexor stretch), and Saddle. Saddle is the most effective for restoring good posture in the sacrum and in the lower part of the spine.

I also again want to remind you that in Yin Yoga poses, you do not need to engage the muscles to hold you in a pose. It is better to align your skeleton in the pose and let Arohan and Awarohan, the breath and props, give you support. Just work toward relaxing your legs, arms, face, and shoulders. Difficult in the beginning, but totally doable.

Set It Up for Your Individual Needs
If you want to add Yin Yoga to your practice, then I advise that you start to integrate this practice with your other practice/training one day a week. Yin Yoga is not a sole yoga practice since you need to stimulate and train the muscluar tissue to receive stability and strength. Yin Yoga is meant to complement a yang practice. However, if you are a professional athlete, then Yin Yoga might be your only yoga practice, since you already get a strong yang practice regularly.

The recommended time to hold a pose should vary by individual. If you find that the general guidelines are not suiting you, explore gently until you find what is apporpriate to you.

My personal advice is to start with holding only three minutes for a couple of weeks to get you used to listening to your body and to work through any limitations or mental blocks. Once you have gained that sensitivity, you can prolong the time to four minutes. Stay within that time lapse for a couple of weeks. For advanced practioners who have practiced well over a couple of years, you can move up to six minutes.

Since you are working with the fascia in your body in this practice, I cannot stress enough the importance of *slowly* coming in and especially out of the pose. Also, do not miss out on the juicy feeling just seconds after coming out of a pose. Sit for a moment, close your eyes, breathe gently, and feel the aftereffects of the pose. It is usually very pleasant. If you move too quickly, you miss out on the endorphin rush and you risk the tissues drawing back together too fast, which can hurt.

Sometimes when you have been in a pose for a couple of minutes you might feel it is impossible to come out of the pose and think you are never going to be able to walk again. But rest assured—you will. Coming out of the pose gently and slowly, followed by some gentle movement and a counterpose, brings it all back to neutral.

Something I like to do is to stimulate the ability to visualize and this is something my students like a lot, too. When you are about to come out of a pose, don't move. First, try to visualize yourself coming out of the pose, how you would move etc., until you come back to neutral. Then let the body follow that inner imaging. You will notice it gives you a whole different sensation and attentiveness.

Also, I often use a "meditation timer." It is an app that is easily downloaded in your smartphone. Or any timer works. The use of a timer is of great benefit I find, since then you can just focus on the sensation, breath, and the meditative practice and not worry about time (quite nice for a change, huh?).

In the poses, use Arohan/Awarohan in line with the breath to start, then as you find a deeper focus, let the breath flow freely and naturally, and just focus on Arohan/Awarohan until your mind quiets. Then you can let that go too. If your mind starts to wander or you start to feel tired, then implement AA again.

In terms of how to integrate Yin Yoga into your existing practice, one recommendation I have is to add some Yin Yoga movements as a start to your regular practice, or as a pre-mediative practice. Yin Yoga also works beautifully as a practice to do just before bed or when you wake up in the morning. It helps to slowly prepare you for the day by adding breath and inner movement, or as a de-stress practice before bedtime, creating better equilibrium in mind, body, and soul.

When you are building your own home practice, or if you are a teacher creating a class for your students, you can work with different inner themes while moving through the practice.

Here are some ideas and recommendations for different focuses during practice that have worked very well for me:

Working with Breath
- Allow the breath to be the anchor for attention, and throughout the practice anchor yourself with the breath, linking the breath to the Arohan/Awarohan kriya.
- Conscious breathing (listening to the sound of the breath/sensing it move inside versus gently stretching the breath)
- The feeling of the breath, how the experience of the body changes at every part of a breath cycle

Physical Sensations
- Without judging and without tampering with the experience, try to let go of "understanding" the experience. Try to just let it be an experience.
- Go deep into the sensation, locate the center of it, its shape, texture, temperature, and changes, breath by breath, moment by moment—without trying to change it, just giving in.
- This can be challenging. Realize that it can be too much, and that sometimes it is better to back off a little than to remain, which can affect the yin qualities of acceptance, trust, and yielding.

Listening/Observation
- Become aware of sounds inside and outside.
- Listen without categorizing sounds as good or bad, pleasant or unpleasant.
- Let sound be just sound.

Thoughts/Feelings
- View the thoughts like events that come and go against a background of alert stillness.
- Follow the thoughts, noting that your thoughts always have a beginning and an end, and that there's a void before the next thought, where we can rest in the open presence.
- Categorize thoughts—use present/past/neutral as a way to understand the habitual and recurring patterns of thought.

- Observe emotions as they come; see if you notice if they are triggered by thoughts or bodily sensations.
- Categorize the feelings—use accept/challenge/neutral as a way to understand the habitual patterns of reaction.
- When working with thoughts as a theme, remember to periodically move the attention back to the body and use Arohan and Awarohan to neutralize and align the energy back to Sattva guna.
- When working with emotions as a theme, be aware that it may be too much. If the experience becomes too intense, come back to the sensations in your body and focus on breathing and surrounding sounds.

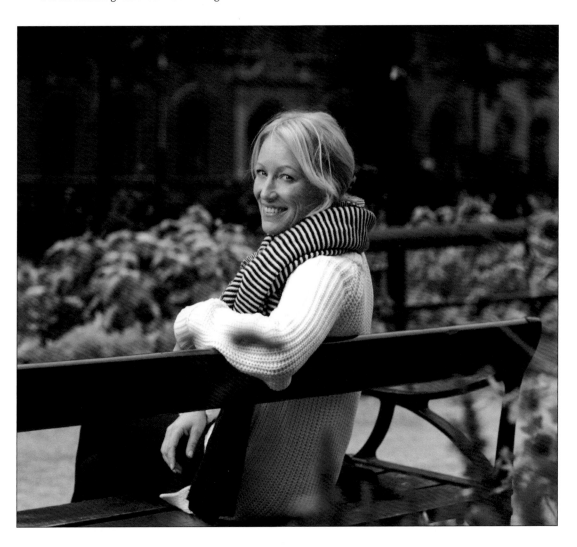

Yin Yoga Flows

Here are some recommended Yin Yoga practice flows you can try. See what fits your needs. These suggested flowing practices will give you 60–75 minutes of yoga. Then in the end, I outline a shorter, 30-minute Yin Yoga practice.

CP= Counterpose

HIP AND LOWER BACK

Start with a yang flow series, working with your breath and integrating Arohan and Awarohan kriya.

1. Child's Pose, tuning in to the breath and sensing the kriya. 8–12 breaths
2. Downward-Facing Dog for 8 breaths
3. Shalabhasana for 8 breaths
4. Child's Pose for 8 breaths
5. Cat-cow flow for 8 breaths
6. Navasana for 8 breaths

Continue with a yin flow series, working with breath and integrating Arohan and Awarohan kriya:
(keep poses 3 to 5 minutes)

7. Child's Pose
CP: Cat-cow 2 times to neutralize
8. Swan/Sleeping Swan—Right side
CP: Cat-cow 2 times to neutralize
9. Swan/Sleeping Swan—Left side
CP: Downward-facing Dog 4 breaths to neutralize
10. Butterfly
CP: Gently sit upright and place your fingertips on the floor behind you and stretch back (no hold). Then gently come to all fours and lay on the belly. Stay and breathe into the belly 4–6 times.

11. Sphinx/Seal (3 min Sphinx, 1 min Seal)

CP: Gently move back to Child's Pose. Then to Cat-cow flow 2-4 times. Come and lay on the back.

12. Happy Baby

13. Reclined twist—Right side

CP: Hug the knees into the chest and rock from side to side gently a couple of times.

14. Reclined twist—Left side

CP: Hug the knees into the chest and rock from side to side gently a couple of times.

15. Savasana for 5 minutes

16. Meditation. Sit upright and find the breath. Integrate Arohan and Awarohan until mind is calm and still. Sit for 5 minutes.

Reground and Namaste.

Sacred Hips

Yin flow series, working with breath and integrating Arohan and Awarohan kriya (keep poses 3–5 minutes)

1. Child's Pose, wide-legged
CP: Cat-cow (no hold, just 4 counts of breath)
2. Saddle
3. Dragon—Right side
CP: Cat-cow (no hold, just 4 counts of breath)
4. Swan/Sleeping Swan—Right side
CP: Cat-cow (no hold, just 4 counts of breath). Come up in Downward-facing dog 4 breaths
5. Dragon—Left side
CP: Cat-cow (no hold, just 4 counts of breath). Come up in Downward-facing dog 4 breaths
6. Swan/Sleeping Swan—Left side
CP: Child's Pose, then on to all fours. Cat-cow (no hold, just 4 counts of breath)
7. Anahatasana
CP: Child's Pose, then on to all fours. Cat-cow (no hold, just 4 counts of breath)
8. Shoelace
CP: Seated twist
9. Caterpillar
CP: Mermaid (right and left side. 4 breaths on each side), then come down to back and hug knees into chest; roll from side to side (no hold, just 4 counts of breath)
10. Savasana 5 minutes
11. Meditation. Sit upright and find your breath. Integrate Arohan and Awarohan until mind is calm and still. Sit for 6–18 minutes. Reground and Namaste.

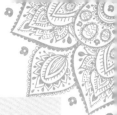

CIRCULATION

Working with breath and integrating Arohan and Awarohan kriya
(keep poses 3–5 minutes)

1. Child's Pose
CP: Cat-cow (no hold, just 4 counts of breath). Come up in Downward-facing dog 4 breaths
2. Seal.
CP: Child's Pose, then on to all fours.
3. Dragon—Right side
CP: Cat-cow (no hold, just 4 counts of breath). Come up in Downward-facing dog 4 breaths
4. Dragon—Left side
CP: Cat-cow (no hold, just 4 counts of breath). Come up in Downward-facing dog 4 breaths
5. Frog
CP: Sit upright and gently open the chest and lean back onto hands.
6. Square pose—Right side
CP: Sit upright and gently open the chest and lean back onto hands.
7. Square pose—Left side
CP: Sit upright and gently open the chest and lean back onto hands. Then come into Mermaid (right and left side. 4 breaths on eash side).
8. Dragonfly with variations
9. Happy Baby
CP: Hug the knees into the chest. Rock from side to side.
10. Savasana 5 minutes
11. Just sit quietly with eyes closed for 3 minutes.

CONTEMPLATION

Working with breath and integrating Arohan and Awarohan kriya
(keep poses 2–5 minutes)
1. Supta padangusthasana sequence—Right side
2. Supta padangusthasana sequence—Left side.
3. Happy Baby
4. Swan on the back—Right side
5. Swan on the back—Left side
CP: Cat-cow (no hold, just 4 counts of breath). Come up in Downward-facing dog 4 breaths.
6. Half-butterfly—Right side
7. Half butterfly—Left side
CP: Cat-cow (no hold, just 4 counts of breath). Come up in Downward-facing dog 4 breaths.
8. Sphinx/Seal
CP: Child's Pose
9. Ankle Stretch
10. Toe Stretch
11. Butterfly
CP: Hug your knees in front of the chest and then roll down vertebra by vertebra to lying down.
12. Snail or Viparita karani
CP: Hug the knees into the chest. Rock from side to side.
13. Savasana 5 minutes
14. Meditation, watching the breath.

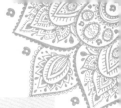

YIN YOGA FLOW SHORT FORM 30 MINUTES

Hold poses 3 minutes

Start with Child's Pose for a couple of breaths, finding inner spaciousness and integrate AA (arohan awarohan).

Then come up to all fours and into cat-cow 4 times.

Then Downward-facing dog 6 breaths. Come back to all fours and into:

1. Butterfly

2. Dragonfly

End with sitting in dragonfly and gently lean side to side in sync with breaths 4 times. Come over onto belly.

3. Cat pulling its tail—Right side

4. Cat pulling its tail—Left side

5. Sphinx

CP: Child's Pose

6. Bananasana—Right side

7. Bananasana—Left side

CP: Reclining twist right/left side—1 minute on each side

8. Savasana 5 minutes

9. Meditation 2 minutes

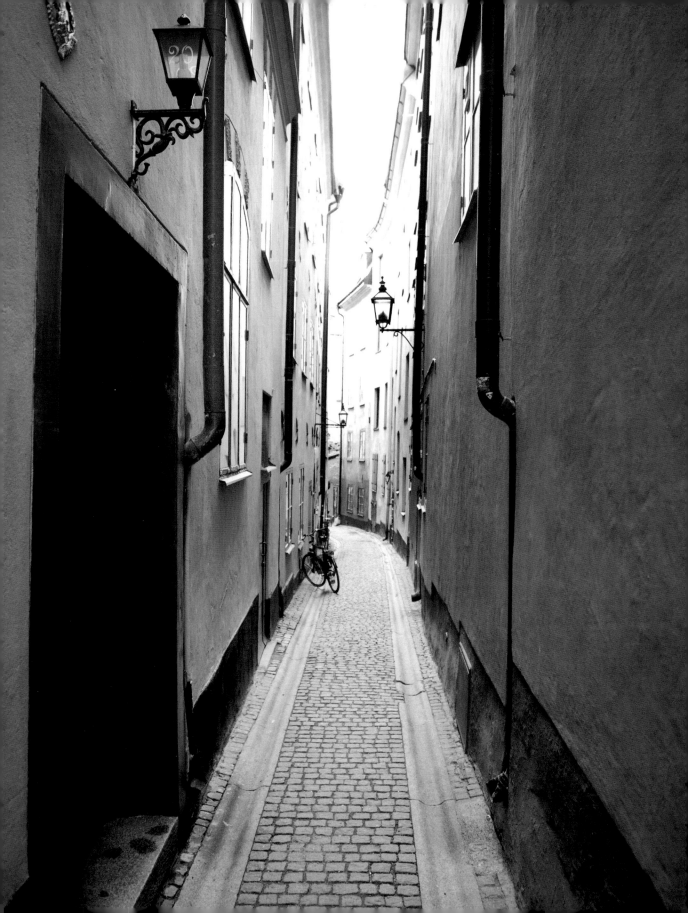

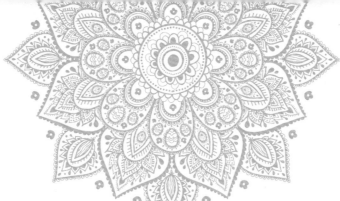

YOGA FROM AN INDIVIDUAL POINT OF VIEW

The subtle body is the gatekeeper between the physical and the spiritual body. Yin Yoga is conditioning training for the subtle body. In order to balance our subtle body, we need to quiet the mind and the nervous system. If we move a lot in yoga practice, it can be quite hard to sense the inner shifts and your limitations—it's easy to wind up listening to your mind rather than your body. Yin Yoga gives you the stillness needed to really listen to the body and to move into spirit, which is all that you are.

Yin Yoga offers an opportunity to strengthen and refine an attitude of openness and trust, allowing a person to be open to what is perhaps perceived as difficult or uncomfortable in body and mind. There is an ongoing practice that is expanding, from the time spent in positions on the yoga mat, into life and everyday life. It provides an opportunity to let things be as they actually are.

FROM AN INDIVIDUAL POINT OF VIEW

Since the lives we live are fast paced and the changes are rapid, we need a practice that helps us to find balance. We are able to reflect more upon ourselves and life.

I think practices like Yoga Nidra, Restorative Yoga, and Yin Yoga will continue to grow more popular the more demanding modern life becomes, since when we hit our speed limit, there is no more acceleration force left, so we are destined to move the opposite way, learning where the brake system is. When we can manuever the gas pedal and put pressure on the brakes, we move towards homeostasis, equilibrium, yoga.

So from an individual standpoint, it is all about being aware of the stressors we have in our life and how they affect us. Maybe we cannot remove them, but what we can do is find alternative ways of relating to them and noting how much impact they have in our life. When we can attain inner stillness for a couple of minutes daily, we can get better perspective on where we are in life and how life plays out both within and without.

HITTING ROAD BUMPS AND LOVELY HIGHS

One day not too long ago, when I was sitting in meditation, I was overwhelmed with the sensation of feeling free in mind, heart, and spirit. It was such a wonderful sensation, and it happens more often than not these days. This inner freedom has not come easily and has been a struggle for me to achieve for many years. Here I was, warm tears streaming down my cheeks. They were tears of hard work, love, and devotion.

Since I started yoga and meditation, I have had my own version of devotion; maybe not true to a long asana practice every day on the mat, but I have not gone one day in almost twenty-one years without checking into my inner world, listening, sensing, and reflecting on what is going on in me and in correlation to the outside world. This reflection has not been free from anxiety, anger, tears, confusion, or other feelings. But I have always felt there is growth happening.

The normative has never been interesting to me. But when one grows up in a middle-sized city in Sweden, the norm is one strives not to stick out. It is hard to realize you are not a part of a normality as a child, teen, and young adult. You become the outlaw, the strange one. I know all too well how it feels to be that person.

Even though I am in a much better state than I was back in my teens, life still happens and there are still aspects of life that are challenging. Today, I strive to find balance in life where family, work, and *me*-time can be better connected and in tune with one another.

After having kids, my practice has changed in that I no longer have the space for a long practice that often. That space I used to grant myself every day is consumed by being a mother, working, and taking care of our home. I still practice daily, aiming for 30–60 minutes a day, but some days 10–20 minutes is all I can make space for.

In terms of choice of practice, I try to adapt to the situation at hand and look at what I need. These days I start the day by observing where I am and through that I conduct a practice based upon trying to attain the lacking quality and aim my practice toward what is needed to balance myself. For example, if I have been sitting writing all day, I usually do a more vigorating practice. And those days I have been up and about, going from place to place, Yin Yoga is my definitive choice since I then need to unwind, destress, and ground myself. The ability to do so has come through practice over years and also for having had a meditation practice for a long time that has helped me to cultivate an attitude to listen inwards.

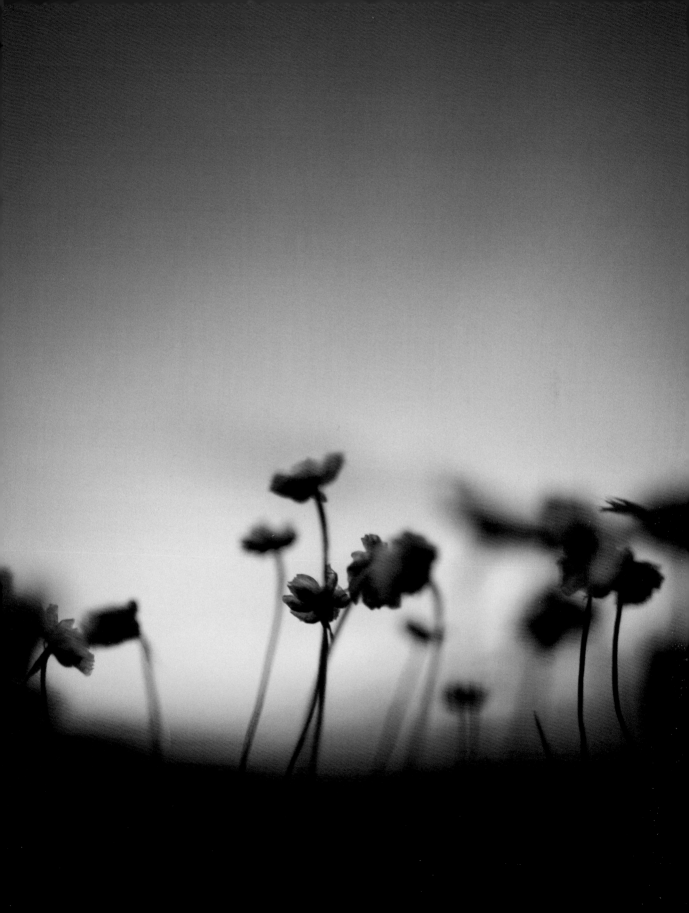

There have been periods in life when I skipped meditation and yoga practice on some days. Those times were some of the most draining and non-balanced periods of my grown-up life. My practice is a way of balancing myself and making me attuned to the flow of life.

DOES ONE NEED A TEACHER?

For as long as I have been a yogi, there has been a discussion in the yoga community about whether a guru/teacher is needed for one's spiritual growth. To me this has been an interesting question all along.

In the beginning of my yoga studies, I struggled with my connection to some of the yoga masters I worked with. I never questioned their knowledge but felt awkward when they wanted to be adored (sometimes worshipped), wanted me to kiss their feet, or treated me disrespectfully because I am a woman. I struggled inside, thinking some days that it was *me*. I felt *I* was wrong, egoistic, attached, not belonging in the yogic community because I had a hard time. I gave it a try, saying to myself that it was not right of me to have opinions about something I had no experience with or knowledge about.

So sometimes I conformed. But after I did it, my gut feeling was that conforming was not for me. However, I have never thought less of anyone else for feeling it was the right thing to do. I envied their feelings of certainty.

Ten years in to my yoga practice, things started to change and I was meeting many inspiring and experienced teachers from different backgrounds in yoga, science, spirituality, and Eastern/Western linkage with a different approach. They were more open, but still very integrated in their own practices. So I studied with many of them, attaining great skills, knowledge, and experience. Their take on yoga appealed to me, telling me the yoga mat and their practice was their guru. I resonated with that perspective a lot, but after a couple of years, new questions arose in me. That perspective about the yoga practice being the guru was starting to feel hollow. I felt that my asana practice could not be all my yoga. And what was it mirroring? Whatever I *wanted*. Not necessarily what I *needed* to keep growing. I started to feel very lonely in my practice, feeling that yoga practice was boring, feeling I should quit yoga all together. The only thing keeping me interested was Savasana and meditation.

Then I started to think, *have I become a lazy yogi? Am I depressed?* Maybe I had reached a point where yoga was not the thing for me anymore. Perhaps something else had to come in and inspire me. I was actually okay with the thought of, if it came to it, not doing yoga anymore. I had gained so much and at that time I was also a mother, feeling that motherhood was so much more important than anything else.

This is when Alan appeared in my life. He said I didn't need more knowledge, but instead needed to learn how to integrate what I had inside me with all my experiences and knowledge about life. He is my friend, mentor, and teacher. He has played a part in my life, making things brighter, lighter, and more clear. He lets me be *me*. So if that is a guru, then he is my guru.

The word "guru" means "shredder of darkness." According to yoga philosophy, the guru comes when you are ready, not when you want. And the yoga philosophy does not say it has to be a man, woman, old person, young person, white, red, or black.

To me, a true teacher is someone who will appear when you need them and are open to them. That teacher will not always say the things you want to hear, but will help you on your spiritual path as a yogi and human. That makes you grow on many levels. You should have an honest and respectful relationship with your guru, one in which all feelings and thoughts are welcome. He or she should not judge you but rather give you tools to deal with your life and imbalances. That makes you evolve as a human.

We all need good teachers and mentors to support us and show us the way to ourselves and the unbound potential that resides within each and every one of us.

Keep practicing and the teacher will come that brings it all together for you. In whatever shape or form.

Thank you for listening and best of wishes on your yogic path onwards.

Namaste.

Oum Shanti,

Ulrica

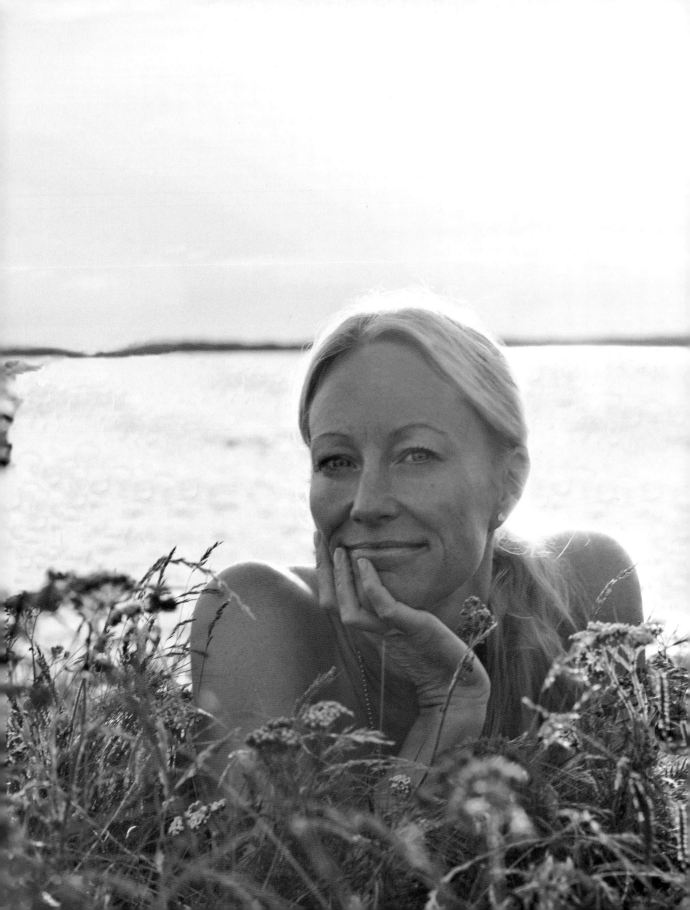

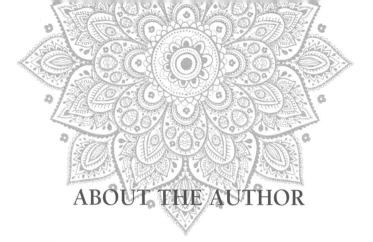

ABOUT THE AUTHOR

Ulrica Norberg (E-RYT 500) is a well-known yogi and writer in Northern Europe with a Masters degree in Human sciences with a major in film, media, and communication. Ulrica's first encounter with yoga was through Zen Buddhist studies in 1994 when she lived in New York City. In the late 1990s she finished her first yoga training in classical Hatha Yoga. That led to even deeper studies in yoga, alignment principles, anatomy, and energetics through various yoga styles and teachers. In early 2002 she discovered Yin Yoga and has since continued her studies in Yin. Ulrica is very intrigued by the mind-body connection and followed her interest in the science of the subtle body to the teachings of ISHTA Yoga. Ulrica is one of ISHTA yoga's senior teachers and is ISHTA yoga's Scandinavian representative. She is currently teaching teacher's trainings, workshops, retreats, conventions, and events for yoga, meditation, and personal growth in addition to writing and coaching.

She was one of the first pioneers of yoga in Scandinavia from 1998 and on, and since then she has taught and coached a vast range of yoga students and trained over 500 yoga teachers in Scandinavia. Ulrica has owned her own studio, travelled around the world several times, made yoga DVDs, and written several books, articles, and audiobooks on yoga, some of which have been translated into different languages. Ulrica is known for her deep knowledge, inquiry, humbleness, and warm approach.

For more information about Ulrica and her workshops, trainings, and events, visit www.ulricanorberg.se.

For more information around ISHTA Yoga and Yoga Master Alan Finger, visit www.ishtayoga.com

BIBLIOGRAPHY

Bjonnes, Ramesh. *Sacred Body, Sacred Spirit: A personal guide to the Wisdom of Yoga and Tantra.* Innerworld Publications, 2012.

Clark, Bernie. *Yin Sights: A Journey into the Philosophy and Practice of Yin Yoga,* White Cloud Press, 2011.

Doidge, Norman. *The Brain that Changes Itself.* Penguin, 2007.

Feurstein, Georg and Jeanine Miller. *The Essence of Yoga,* Inner Traditions, 2014.

Finger, Alan, ISHTA YOGA LLC. *The Teachers Training Manuals 200+300* hr

Finger, Alan and Al Binghan. *Introduction to Yoga,* Three Rivers Press, 2000.

Gerst, Cole. *Buckminster Fuller: Poet of Geometry*, Option-G, 2013.

Grilley, Paul. *Yin Yoga,* White Cloud Press, 2012.

Judkins, Rod. *Change Your Mind,* Hardie Grant Books, 2013.

Muktibodhananda, Swami. *Hathayoga Pradipika,* Yoga Publications Trust, 1998.

Myers, Thomas W. *Anatomy Trains: Myofascial Meridians for Manual and Movement Therapists*, Churchill Livingstone, 2008.

Perski, Alexander. *Ur Balans*, Albert Bonniers förlag, 2006.

Powers, Sarah. *Insight Yoga*, Shambala Publications Inc., 2013.

Sapolsky, Robert M. *Why Zebras Don't get Ulcers,* Holt, 2004.

Satchidananda, Swami. *Yoga Sutras of Patanjali*, Integral Yoga Publications, 2012.

Schleip, Robert (PhD) et al. *Fascia: The Tensional Network of the Human Body*, Churchill Livingstone, 2012.

Singh, Gagandeep and Raghu Ananthanarayanan. *Organizational Development and Alignment: The Tensegrity Mandala Framework*, Sage Publications, 2013.

Yogananda, Paramhansa. *Autobiography of a Yogi.* Self-Realization Fellowship, 1998.

Yogananda, Paramhansa. *Demystifying Patanjali: The Yoga Sutras*, Crystal Clarity, 2013.

Websites:

www.ulricanorberg.se
www.Ishtayoga.com
www.ishtayoga.se

YIN YOGA JOURNAL

YIN YOGA JOURNAL

YIN YOGA JOURNAL

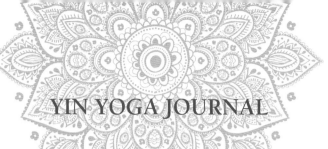

YIN YOGA JOURNAL

YIN YOGA JOURNAL

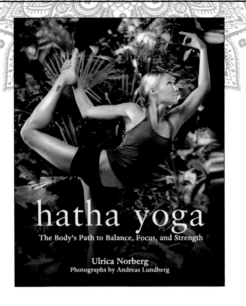

Hatha yoga

The Body's Path to Balance, Focus, and Strength

by Ulrica Norberg

For the 16.5 million yoga practitioners in America, Swedish yoga instructor Ulrica Norberg's fresh look at Hatha yoga ("the way of the body") will be a perfect entrée to the art of exercising to produce a strong mind and a harmonious soul. Focusing on pacing, not perfection, Norberg explains proper breathing and asanas, poses developed to increase consciousness, relaxation, strength, and concentration. Throughout, she maintains a thoughtful balance between philosophy and instruction, and offers step-by-step directions and wisdom for personal and communal well-being. Lavishly illustrated with gorgeous full-color photographs, *Hatha yoga* is sure to inspire beginning and advanced yoga practitioners alike. 100 color photographs

$14.95 Paperback • ISBN: 978-1-60239-218-2

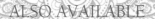

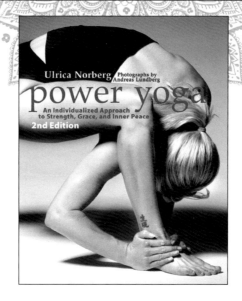

Power Yoga, 2nd Edition

An Individualized Approach to Strength, Grace, and Inner Peace

by Ulrica Norberg

Norberg believes yoga can aid us in developing our own life philosophies through a synthesis of Eastern ideology and self-reflection. Her book *Power Yoga* is at once a testament to the beauty and grace of yoga and a how-to guide that explains practice and form.

Norberg takes readers through the elements of yoga and the basic movements and techniques specific to power yoga. Filled with beautiful full-color photographs illustrating sun-salutations (the basis of power yoga exercises), numerous asanas (poses), and meditation techniques, her book is useful for all levels of instruction and inspiration. This is one of the few practical yoga books that truly expresses the joy, physicality, and temperament of yoga, which has become a passion for so many Americans—young and old and men and women alike. 150 color photographs

$14.95 Paperback • ISBN: 978-1-61608-172-0